Marijuana

OTHER BOOKS OF RELATED INTEREST

Marijuana

Louise I. Gerdes, *Book Editor*

Daniel Leone, *President*
Bonnie Szumski, *Publisher*
Scott Barbour, *Managing Editor*
Brenda Stalcup, *Series Editor*

Contemporary Issues
Companion

Greenhaven Press, Inc., San Diego, CA

Every effort has been made to trace the owners of copyrighted material. The articles in this volume may have been edited for content, length, and/or reading level. The titles have been changed to enhance the editorial purpose. Those interested in locating the original source will find the complete citation on the first page of each article.

Library of Congress Cataloging-in-Publication Data

Marijuana / Louise I. Gerdes, book editor.
    p. cm. — (Contemporary issues companion)
    Includes bibliographical references and index.
    ISBN 0-7377-0834-4 (pbk. : alk. paper) —
ISBN 0-7377-0835-2 (lib. : alk. paper)
    1. Marijuana. 2. Marijuana—Therapeutic use. 3. Marijuana—Law and legislation. I. Gerdes, Louise. II. Series.

HV5822.M3 M267 2002
362.29'5—dc21   2001040744
                                                 CIP

© 2002 by Greenhaven Press, Inc.
10911 Technology Place, San Diego, CA 92127

Printed in the U.S.A.

CONTENTS

FOREWORD

In the news, on the streets, and in neighborhoods, individuals are confronted with a variety of social problems. Such problems may affect people directly: A young woman may struggle with depression, suspect a friend of having bulimia, or watch a loved one battle cancer. And even the issues that do not directly affect her private life—such as religious cults, domestic violence, or legalized gambling—still impact the larger society in which she lives. Discovering and analyzing the complexities of issues that encompass communal and societal realms as well as the world of personal experience is a valuable educational goal in the modern world.

Effectively addressing social problems requires familiarity with a constantly changing stream of data. Becoming well informed about today's controversies is an intricate process that often involves reading myriad primary and secondary sources, analyzing political debates, weighing various experts' opinions—even listening to firsthand accounts of those directly affected by the issue. For students and general observers, this can be a daunting task because of the sheer volume of information available in books, periodicals, on the evening news, and on the Internet. Researching the consequences of legalized gambling, for example, might entail sifting through congressional testimony on gambling's societal effects, examining private studies on Indian gaming, perusing numerous websites devoted to Internet betting, and reading essays written by lottery winners as well as interviews with recovering compulsive gamblers. Obtaining valuable information can be time-consuming—since it often requires researchers to pore over numerous documents and commentaries before discovering a source relevant to their particular investigation.

Greenhaven's Contemporary Issues Companion series seeks to assist this process of research by providing readers with useful and pertinent information about today's complex issues. Each volume in this anthology series focuses on a topic of current interest, presenting informative and thought-provoking selections written from a wide variety of viewpoints. The readings selected by the editors include such diverse sources as personal accounts and case studies, pertinent factual and statistical articles, and relevant commentaries and overviews. This diversity of sources and views, found in every Contemporary Issues Companion, offers readers a broad perspective in one convenient volume.

In addition, each title in the Contemporary Issues Companion series is designed especially for young adults. The selections included in every volume are chosen for their accessibility and are expertly edited in consideration of both the reading and comprehension levels of the audience. The structure of the anthologies also enhances accessibility. An introductory essay places each issue in context and provides helpful facts such as historical background or current statistics and legislation that pertain to the topic. The chapters that follow organize the material and focus on specific aspects of the book's topic. Every essay is introduced by a brief summary of its main points and biographical information about the author. These summaries aid in comprehension and can also serve to direct readers to material of immediate interest and need. Finally, a comprehensive index allows readers to efficiently scan and locate content.

The Contemporary Issues Companion series is an ideal launching point for research on a particular topic. Each anthology in the series is composed of readings taken from an extensive gamut of resources, including periodicals, newspapers, books, government documents, the publications of private and public organizations, and Internet websites. In these volumes, readers will find factual support suitable for use in reports, debates, speeches, and research papers. The anthologies also facilitate further research, featuring a book and periodical bibliography and a list of organizations to contact for additional information.

A perfect resource for both students and the general reader, Greenhaven's Contemporary Issues Companion series is sure to be a valued source of current, readable information on social problems that interest young adults. It is the editors' hope that readers will find the Contemporary Issues Companion series useful as a starting point to formulate their own opinions about and answers to the complex issues of the present day.

INTRODUCTION

California author and publisher Peter McWilliams was diagnosed with both AIDS and cancer in 1996. Under his doctor's supervision, McWilliams began to smoke marijuana to quell the nausea caused by the combination drug therapy he took to keep the AIDS virus at undetectable levels. He believed that he was doing so legally under California's Proposition 215. This state law, passed in 1996, prohibits the prosecution of those who use marijuana for medical reasons.

In July 1998, however, McWilliams was arrested and tried for collaborating in the illegal growth of marijuana plants. He was prosecuted under a federal law prohibiting the cultivation of marijuana, and the federal judge would not allow him to plead his defense under California's Proposition 215, stating that the federal legislation superseded the state law. McWilliams was found guilty, and although he was allowed to serve his sentence at home, his urine was regularly tested for marijuana: If any traces were found in his system, he would be returned to prison. On June 14, 2000, racked by nausea, McWilliams died by choking on his own vomit—a death that some people believed might have been prevented if McWilliams had been allowed to continue controlling his nausea with marijuana.

Whether marijuana is effective as a treatment for nausea and other medical problems is a hotly contested issue. A significant population of seriously ill patients report that smoking marijuana appears to alleviate the debilitating side effects of their illnesses, including the nausea associated with chemotherapy, the loss of appetite that comes with AIDS, the spasms that accompany spastic disorders and spinal cord injuries, and the chronic pain of other diseases and injuries. "Thousands of patients . . . report they have obtained striking relief from these devastating symptoms by smoking marijuana," Jerome P. Kasirer, then editor in chief of the *New England Journal of Medicine*, wrote in a January 30, 1997, editorial. Based on the testimony of such patients and their own clinical experience, a number of physicians and scientists have concluded that marijuana does indeed have proven medical properties. Furthermore, they note, a few medical studies—such as those that show marijuana to be helpful in the treatment of glaucoma—bolster these patients' claims.

On the other hand, many nationally recognized experts in the scientific community dispute the theory that marijuana has measurable medical benefits. They point out that this belief is primarily founded on personal testimonies from patients rather than on dispassionate experimentation and controlled clinical studies. According to Billy Martin, chief of pharmacology at the Medical College of Virginia, "We lack evidence that there is something unique about marijuana, other than an impressive number of anecdotal reports." These critics also express concern over the very act of smoking marijuana, which they warn can lead to respiratory disease and possibly even cancer. Organizations such as the American Cancer Society, the National Sclerosis Association, and the American Glaucoma Association have concluded that smoking marijuana is not safe and therefore cannot be considered an effective medical treatment. Moreover, both the Food and Drug Administration (FDA) and the U.S. Public Health Service have rejected the smoking of crude marijuana as a safe and effective delivery method.

Nevertheless, the medicinal use of marijuana—whether administered by smoking or some other method—has continued to gain acceptance not only in the medical community but also among the general public. In an analysis of forty-seven national drug policy surveys conducted between 1978 and 1997, researchers at the Harvard School of Public Health found that more than 60 percent of the public currently supported "legalized use of marijuana for medical purposes." In fact, several states have followed California's lead in decriminalizing the use of medical marijuana: By the year 2000, Alaska, Arizona, Colorado, Hawaii, Maine, Nevada, Oregon, and Washington had all passed medical marijuana initiatives.

Notwithstanding the passage of these state laws, however, the federal government continues to consider marijuana a hazardous and illegal drug, classifying it as a Schedule I drug. Federal law defines Schedule I drugs as those that have a high potential for abuse, no currently accepted medical application, and a lack of acceptable safety for use under medical supervision. Since federal legislation prohibits the use of marijuana for any reason, federal law enforcement agencies have no way in which to distinguish the cultivation and distribution of marijuana for medical use from the general trafficking of marijuana as a recreational drug. Under federal law, people like McWilliams who are caught growing marijuana face a mandatory minimum sentence of ten years to life. States can pass initiatives intended to protect patients who use medical marijuana under a physician's supervision, but these state laws may not stand up in court against the federal laws that criminalize all use and cultivation of the drug.

For the most part, both sides of the controversy over medical marijuana agree that further research is necessary to definitively prove or disprove the drug's effectiveness in treating various illnesses. To this end, in February 1997 the White House's Office of National Drug Control Policy commissioned the National Institute on Drug Abuse (NIDA) to assemble a panel to review the scientific evidence on the medicinal use of marijuana. The panel conducted an eighteen-month investigation of marijuana's benefits and risks through a series of public hearings and an exhaustive study of current research. During the public hearings in California, Louisiana, and Washington, D.C., the panel of scientists heard the testimony of experts from both sides of the medical marijuana debate and listened to patients who use marijuana for a wide range of ailments.

In March 1999, the National Academy of Sciences' Institute of Medicine (IOM) released a report entitled *Marijuana and Medicine: Assessing the Science Base*, which detailed the findings of the panel's review of scientific evidence concerning the potential health benefits and risks of marijuana. However, the IOM report did not come down squarely on either side of the medical marijuana debate, as both supporters and opponents had hoped. On one hand, for example, the report revealed that some of the cannabinoid substances found in smoked marijuana have "potential therapeutic value . . . moderately well-suited for certain conditions, such as chemotherapy-induced nausea and vomiting and AIDS wasting." On the other hand, the report found smoking to be an unsafe delivery system, recommending that medical marijuana be used only under extremely limited conditions.

The IOM report indicated that further research was needed to clearly determine the medical efficacy of marijuana. Many proponents of medical marijuana claim that the federal government and its agencies hinder such research by making it nearly impossible to legally obtain marijuana for clinical studies. They contend that since the government opposes the use of medical marijuana, it purposely withholds the plant from researchers who might be able to prove marijuana's medicinal value. According to the Marijuana Policy Project, "The National Institute on Drug Abuse—the only legal source of marijuana for research—has been blocking clinical trials by refusing to provide marijuana to FDA-approved studies." However, NIDA denies allegations that it has withheld marijuana for research, and in 2000 the institute supplied researchers with the marijuana needed for scientifically rigorous studies. That same year, the Center for Medicinal Cannabis Research was established at the University of California at San Diego to provide $9 million over several years to California researchers.

Meanwhile, advocates of medical marijuana suffered a legal setback in the spring of 2001. After the passage of California's Proposition 215 in 1996, organizations known as cannabis clubs were formed to provide marijuana to seriously ill patients. Opponents of medical marijuana claimed that the clubs sold the drug in violation of federal laws prohibiting the distribution of marijuana. In May 1998, the Oakland Cannabis Buyers' Cooperative (OCBC) was enjoined by the district court from distributing marijuana in violation of the Controlled Substances Act. The OCBC appealed to the Ninth Circuit Court, which reversed the earlier decision, stating that the OCBC could supply marijuana to people with serious medical conditions for whom legal alternatives to marijuana do not work or cause intolerable side effects. Soon thereafter, the U.S. Supreme Court issued an emergency order barring the distribution of marijuana by the OCBC until it could consider the merits of the case.

On May 14, 2001, the Supreme Court reversed the circuit court's decision, ruling that California's cannabis clubs could not legally distribute marijuana as a "medical necessity" for seriously ill patients. In addition, the Court refused to carve out a medical necessity exception to the federal law that prohibits the distribution of marijuana. According to many observers, this decision effectively invalidated California's 1996 medical marijuana initiative. However, four of the Court's more moderate members issued a separate opinion emphasizing that the ruling applied only to the cannabis clubs and did not necessarily deprive patients and their primary caregivers of the medical necessity defense against federal prosecution.

However it is interpreted, the Supreme Court decision does not mark the end of the medical marijuana debate. Since the decision was handed down, the state legislatures of both Maryland and Massachusetts have introduced bills that, if passed, would protect patients who use medical marijuana from arrest and prosecution. Moreover, in June 2001, the American Medical Association voted to rescind its position opposing medical marijuana, choosing to take a neutral stance on "compassionate use." Conversely, many in the scientific and medical community continue to question the medicinal effectiveness of marijuana, and the U.S. Department of Justice's position remains firm— marijuana is a dangerous drug with no proven medical benefits. For all those involved in the medical marijuana debate, the fight is far from over.

The controversy surrounding the medical use of marijuana is just one aspect of a larger debate over whether the drug should be legalized. Some activists maintain that marijuana should be legal not only for medicinal purposes but also for recreational use. Others oppose outright legalization but promote decriminalization, claiming that the legal penalties for the cultivation, sale, and use of marijuana are too severe. Opponents of marijuana support strong legislative measures and strict penalties; they argue that legalization of any kind would not only increase marijuana use but also lead to the abuse of harder drugs. *Marijuana: Contemporary Issues Companion* presents these views and many others in articles ranging from scientific surveys to editorials to personal accounts. By examining all sides of the marijuana debate, the following chapters offer a broad overview of this controversial issue.

CHAPTER 1

THE EFFECTS OF MARIJUANA

THE HARMFUL EFFECTS OF MARIJUANA

George Biernson

According to George Biernson, many young people are led to believe that marijuana is no more harmful than the alcohol their parents drink. However, Biernson states, alcohol dissolves in the blood and leaves the body quickly, whereas the active ingredient found in marijuana, tetrahydrocannabinol (THC), is stored in the body fat and is slowly released into the bloodstream over longer periods of time. As a result, the author claims, users experience a constant state of sedation and build up a tolerance to marijuana that often prompts them to experiment with stronger drugs. Furthermore, he reveals, research shows that marijuana damages the brain, the chromosomes, and the immune and reproductive systems. Biernson is an electronics systems engineer who used his expertise in kinetics to study the storage of THC in the human body.

Marijuana is very deceptive because it is extremely slow acting.

Very little of its active ingredient, tetrahydrocannabinol (THC), has reached the brain at the time of the "high." Hence the drug appears to the user to be mild.

However, the user does not realize that it has an appreciable effect on his body for over a month.

About 40% of the THC is stored in the body fat and is then slowly released into the blood over many weeks. Each joint adds to the supply of THC that the body is storing, thereby increasing the level of it in the blood. When a person smokes regularly, the THC in his blood is sufficient to sedate him all the time.

Marijuana Is Not Harmless

As they experiment, kids play with pot because they hear from many sources that it is no more harmful than alcohol. Therefore, they reason, "If my parents can drink alcohol, I can smoke pot." As they experiment, the pot appears to be mild, and so they try it again and again. The THC builds up in their bodies and it steadily drags them into a state of continual sedation. Their minds become confused, and their drug use escalates. They usually start drinking alcohol heavily also. In time their brains become so confused that many graduate to the use of cocaine and heroin, drugs they would never have taken before being caught in the marijuana trap.

It is often claimed that marijuana is not harmful because it is not an "addictive drug." The basis for this claim is that physical withdrawal symptoms are mild when one abruptly stops smoking it. However, the reason for mild withdrawal symptoms is that the body has been storing the THC in the body fat and has its own supply of THC.

Prior to 1970, most of the pot had about 1% THC or less, and the best stuff had 3%. Because of the enormous demand for marijuana since the 1960s, a strong effort was expended to develop new varieties. Today, practically all of the street pot has about 12%, and some has as much as 25%. Thus the marijuana available today is about ten times as potent as in the 1960s.

Brain Damage

Dr. Robert Heath of Tulane Medical School did extensive studies of the effect of marijuana on the brains of monkeys. He was world-renowned for his research on the brain, and he was the head of the departments of psychiatry and neurology at five hospitals in the New Orleans area.

A typical experiment performed by Dr. Heath was to allow a monkey to smoke the equivalent of a human's smoking two joints of pot per day containing 2.5% THC, five days per week for six months. The monkey was allowed to recover for six months and then was killed. Brain waves were measured from electrodes embedded in the brain. The brain waves had become severely distorted after two months of smoking, and remained severely distorted until the monkey was killed.

The cells in the brain, which were examined under an electron microscope, showed serious damage, particularly in a deep part of the brain called the limbic system, which is the center of emotion. All of the brain cells of the limbic region showed strong structural changes. For monkeys that smoked only 40% of this amount, the damage was much less but was still observable.

The level of marijuana use by the monkey is equivalent to the smoking of two joints per week of modern pot with 12% THC, by a teenager weighing 130 pounds. We can expect serious long-term brain damage from this level of marijuana use. We can also expect detectable brain damage in a teenager smoking half this level, i.e., one joint of 12% THC per week.

About 1980, this monumental research was cancelled by the National Institute of Drug Abuse, which is the U.S. federal agency that sponsors research on drugs. It buried the results of this research.

Other Damage to the Body

Regular marijuana use at levels generally assumed to be moderate can seriously damage the chromosomes, the immune system, the hormones, the reproductive system, the sex organs, the sex drive, the lungs, and, as we have seen, the brain. Some of it is as follows:

• It causes severe damage to the T-lymphocytes, which are the primary white blood cells associated with the immune defenses of the body, according to studies performed in the early 1970s. The damage to these cells caused by other drugs such as alcohol, cocaine, and heroin is insignificant in comparison to marijuana. These are the blood cells of the immune system that are primarily damaged by AIDS.

• The chromosomes of mice are also severely damaged, according to studies performed by Dr. Susan Dalterio of the University of Texas. Severe abnormalities were caused in newborn mice from use by the grandfather, even with no marijuana use by the grandmother, father or mother.

• The effect on the reproductive system can be severe. Regular use of the drug by children who have not reached puberty can retard and even permanently inhibit sexual maturity. Its use can destroy the sperm and egg cells and thereby cause sterility. Pot smoking is particularly harmful to girls because their ovaries do not produce new egg cells.

Economic Influences

If the scientific case against marijuana is so strong, why are there such strong beliefs that it is relatively harmless? The primary answer is that powerful economic forces are working to keep the marijuana issue confused.

Hundreds of billions of dollars are being made from cocaine and heroin each year. We can expect that much of this money is being spent every year in disguised advertising and influence to help support the trade. As long as the kids believe that marijuana is relatively harmless, many of them will play around with it, and this generates a steady supply of cocaine and heroin addicts.

We were making progress when the National Institute of Drug Abuse supported excellent research on marijuana in the 1970s. However, new leadership took control about 1980, and all of this was cancelled. Since then, the Institute has not supported any significant responsible research on marijuana. In 1988 the United States government sponsored the White House Conference for a Drug-Free America which recommended that an independent evaluation of the National Institute on Drug Abuse be conducted.

No action was ever taken on this recommendation. Nevertheless our federal government spends billions of dollars every year in a fruitless War on Drugs, which attempts to keep drugs from entering our country.

The Medical Use of Marijuana

The attempts to legalize it for medicinal purposes are an indirect means of achieving the total legalization of the drug. Even more important, the message that is being spread concerning the medical use of marijuana is very effective advertising to convince kids that marijuana is not very harmful. This advertising is many, many times more effective than the "Joe Camel" ads by the tobacco companies, which lure kids to smoke tobacco.

We have seen that marijuana severely damages the immune system. How then can we justify telling unfortunate AIDS patients that they should smoke marijuana to lessen their pains? Instead we should be shouting, "With your weak immune systems, you should consider marijuana to be the worst form of poison."

It's also being used by some cancer patients, but it's just as bad for them. Although chemotherapy can cause severe nausea and THC is very effective in combating nausea, the last thing a cancer chemotherapy patient needs is marijuana, which would weaken his immune system further.

There is probably enough common sense in our country to keep us from falling for the phony plea to legalize medical marijuana. However, the primary harm from this campaign is its associated propaganda. This propaganda is convincing countless youngsters that marijuana is harmless.

The Fat Solubility of THC

The reason that marijuana is much more dangerous than alcohol is because the alcohol is water-soluble and it dissolves readily into the blood. It is absorbed from the stomach and stays in the blood until it is metabolized by the liver. The blood carries the alcohol to the brain, where it performs its numbing effect.

In contrast, the THC that is found in marijuana is not soluble in water and so cannot dissolve in the blood.

When a person smokes marijuana, no more than 25% of the THC is absorbed into the blood. About 40% of the THC that enters the body is stored deeply in body fat. The fat releases the THC into the blood with a half-life of one week, which means that if a person stops smoking pot it takes one week for the stored THC to drop to 1/2, two weeks to drop to 1/4, etc. Every week the THC is stored in the fat, it decreases by one-half.

The blood in the brain is separated from the main blood supply by the blood-brain barrier, which is a sieve that helps to protect the brain from toxic substances. Since the THC molecules stick to this sieve, they pass through the blood-brain barrier very slowly. This delays the flow of THC to the brain. By the time an appreciable amount of THC has worked its way through the blood-brain barrier, there is little THC left in the blood. Consequently the peak concentration of THC in the brain blood is very small. It is only 1/2 of one percent of the initial THC concentration in the main blood supply.

At the time of the "high," the peak concentration of THC in the blood of the brain is about 1/1000 of the THC in the marijuana joint, spread over the blood supply of the body.

THC is extremely potent. It is one million times more potent than alcohol. Marijuana appears to be mild because THC acts very slowly, over a period of many weeks.

The more often one smokes marijuana, the more THC is stored in the body fat. The THC stored in body fat is released steadily into the blood. Although the blood-brain barrier delays the flow of this THC to the brain, it does not reduce the amount of THC in the brain because the fat releases THC slowly and steadily. When a person smokes one marijuana joint per day, the peak change of THC concentration in the blood of his brain after smoking a joint is only 3 times the steady THC concentration. He builds up tolerance to the steady THC level, and so he does not feel a strong "high" when smoking a single joint.

The regular pot smoker is constantly sedated from the steady THC level, and so he sinks into a state of continual sedation. His mind becomes confused, he becomes lazy and sloppy, and he has a strong urge to feel "high." Since he is tolerant to the steady THC in his blood, he often turns to other drugs to get "high." Nevertheless, he continues to smoke pot as he takes the other drugs, because smoking marijuana makes him "feel good all the time."

One of the drugs that marijuana smokers take frequently is alcohol. Those who smoke pot usually drink much more alcohol and drink much harder than those who do not. Normally a young person becomes sick and vomits when he drinks excessive alcohol. However THC strongly inhibits nausea, and so a young pot smoker can easily consume a lethal dose of alcohol without vomiting. For someone who does not smoke pot, it normally takes many years of hard alcohol drinking before one builds up sufficient alcohol tolerance to hold down a lethal dose of alcohol without vomiting.

Our society is deeply troubled by the smoking of cigarettes by teen-agers. Yet nobody seems concerned that nearly as many teenagers smoke marijuana as smoke cigarettes. How do you convince a teenager to stop smoking cigarettes when he is smoking pot?

Relationship to Crime

Individuals directly involved in prosecuting criminals are well aware of the strong relation between crime and drug abuse. One district attorney stated that most of the criminals in our jails were so confused by drugs when they committed their crimes they cannot even remember the crimes for which they are bring punished. Marijuana is the seed from which the scourge of drug abuse grows. If we stop the marijuana, we will stop the rest of the drug abuse, and with it the crime.

The marijuana presently being smoked by our kids is ten times as potent as in the 1960s. When we realize how much marijuana is being used by our teenagers, and how extremely potent it is, it is frightening to think of the damage that this marijuana must be doing to the brains of these innocent children. None of us should be surprised by the violence in our schools today.

Myths About the Harmful Effects of Marijuana

Paul Hager

Many claims against marijuana are either false or misleading, writes Paul Hager in the following selection. Hager reveals, for example, that the Partnership for a Drug-Free America fabricated evidence that marijuana use flattens brainwaves. Moreover, he asserts, in several studies—such as those that claim marijuana damages the reproductive system—animals were given extremely high doses of the drug, and researchers have not been able to duplicate similar results in human beings. Other claims about marijuana are true, Hager concedes, but he argues that they are often interpreted in misleading ways: For example, although marijuana does impair short-term memory, the effect is not permanent. Hager, who advocates the legalization of marijuana and other drugs, is a software engineer in Indianapolis, Indiana, and an active member of the Libertarian Party.

1. Marijuana causes brain damage.

The most celebrated study that claims to show brain damage is the rhesus monkey study of Dr. Robert Heath, done in the late 1970s. This study was reviewed by a distinguished panel of scientists sponsored by the Institute of Medicine and the National Academy of Sciences. Their results were published under the title *Marijuana and Health* in 1982. Heath's work was sharply criticized for its insufficient sample size (only four monkeys), its failure to control experimental bias, and the misidentification of normal monkey brain structure as "damaged." Actual studies of human populations of marijuana users have shown no evidence of brain damage. For example, two studies from 1977, published in the *Journal of the American Medical Association (JAMA)* showed no evidence of brain damage in heavy users of marijuana. That same year, the American Medical Association (AMA) officially came out in favor of decriminalizing marijuana. That's not the sort of thing you'd expect if the AMA thought marijuana damaged the brain.

Reprinted, with permission, from "Marijuana Myths," by Paul Hager, *The Libertarian Corner*, www.cs.indiana.edu/hyplan/hagerp/drugwar.html, 1996.

2. Marijuana damages the reproductive system.

This claim is based chiefly on the work of Dr. Gabriel Nahas, who experimented with tissue (cells) isolated in petri dishes, and the work of researchers who dosed animals with near-lethal amounts of cannabinoids (i.e., the intoxicating part of marijuana). Nahas' generalizations from his petri dishes to human beings have been rejected by the scientific community as being invalid. In the case of the animal experiments, the animals that survived their ordeal returned to normal within 30 days of the end of the experiment. Studies of actual human populations have failed to demonstrate that marijuana adversely affects the reproductive system.

3. Marijuana is a "gateway" drug—it leads to hard drugs.

This is one of the more persistent myths. A real world example of what happens when marijuana is readily available can be found in Holland. The Dutch partially legalized marijuana in the 1970s. Since then, hard drug use—heroin and cocaine—have *declined* substantially. If marijuana really were a gateway drug, one would have expected use of hard drugs to have gone up, not down. This apparent "negative gateway" effect has also been observed in the United States. Studies done in the early 1970s showed a negative correlation between use of marijuana and use of alcohol. A 1993 Rand Corporation study that compared drug use in states that had decriminalized marijuana versus those that had not, found that where marijuana was more available—the states that had decriminalized—hard drug abuse as measured by emergency room episodes decreased. In short, what science and actual experience tell us is that marijuana tends to substitute for the much more dangerous hard drugs like alcohol, cocaine, and heroin.

4. Marijuana suppresses the immune system.

Like the studies claiming to show damage to the reproductive system, this myth is based on studies where animals were given extremely high—in many cases, near-lethal—doses of cannabinoids. These results have never been duplicated in human beings.

5. Marijuana is much more dangerous than tobacco.

Smoked marijuana contains about the same amount of carcinogens as does an equivalent amount of tobacco. It should be remembered, however, that a heavy tobacco smoker consumes much more tobacco than a heavy marijuana smoker consumes marijuana. This is because smoked tobacco, with a 90% addiction rate, is the most addictive of all drugs while marijuana is less addictive than caffeine. Two other factors are important. The first is that paraphernalia laws directed against marijuana users make it difficult to smoke safely. These laws make water pipes and bongs, which filter some of the carcinogens out of the smoke, illegal and, hence, unavailable. The second is that, if marijuana were legal, it would be more economical to have cannabis drinks like bhang (a traditional drink in the Middle East) or tea which are totally non-carcinogenic. This is in stark contrast with "smoke-less" tobacco products like snuff which can cause cancer of the mouth and throat. When all of these facts are taken together, it can be clearly seen that the reverse is true: marijuana is much *safer* than tobacco.

6. Legal marijuana would cause carnage on the highways.

Although marijuana, when used to intoxication, does impair perfor-mance in a manner similar to alcohol, actual studies of the effect of marijuana on the automobile accident rate suggest that it poses *less* of a hazard than alcohol. When a random sample of fatal accident vic-tims was studied, it was initially found that marijuana was associated with *relatively* as many accidents as alcohol. In other words, the num-ber of accident victims intoxicated on marijuana relative to the num-ber of marijuana users in society gave a ratio similar to that for acci-dent victims intoxicated on alcohol relative to the total number of alcohol users. However, a closer examination of the victims revealed that around 85% of the people intoxicated on marijuana *were also intoxicated on alcohol*. For people only intoxicated on marijuana, the rate was much lower than for alcohol alone. This finding has been supported by other research using completely different methods. For example, an economic analysis of the effects of decriminalization on marijuana usage found that states that had reduced penalties for mar-ijuana possession experienced a rise in marijuana use and a decline in alcohol use with the result that fatal highway accidents decreased. This would suggest that, far from causing "carnage," legal marijuana might actually save lives.

7. Marijuana "flattens" human brainwaves.

This is an out-and-out lie perpetrated by the Partnership for a Drug-Free America. A few years ago, they ran a TV ad that purported to show, first, a normal human brainwave, and second, a flat brainwave from a 14-year-old "on marijuana." When researchers called up the TV networks to complain about this commercial, the Partnership had to pull it from the air. It seems that the Partnership faked the flat "marijuana brainwave." In reality, marijuana has the effect of slightly *increasing* alpha wave activity. Alpha waves are associated with medi-tative and relaxed states which are, in turn, often associated with human creativity.

8. Marijuana is more potent today than in the past.

This myth is the result of bad data. The researchers who made the claim of increased potency used as their baseline the THC content of marijuana seized by police in the early 1970s. Poor storage of this marijuana in unair-conditioned evidence rooms caused it to deteriorate and decline in potency before any chemical assay was performed. Contemporaneous, independent assays of unseized "street" marijuana from the early 1970s showed a potency equivalent to that of modern "street" marijuana. Actually, the most potent form of this drug that was generally available was sold legally in the 1920s and 1930s by the pharmaceutical company Smith-Klein under the name "American Cannabis."

9. Marijuana impairs short-term memory.

This is true but misleading. Any impairment of short-term memory disappears when one is no longer under the influence of marijuana. Often, the short-term memory effect is paired with a reference to Dr. Heath's poor rhesus monkeys to imply that the condition is permanent.

10. Marijuana lingers in the body like DDT.

This is also true but misleading. Cannabinoids are fat soluble as are innumerable nutrients and, yes, some poisons like DDT. For example, the essential nutrient, Vitamin A, is fat soluble but one never hears people who favor marijuana prohibition making this comparison.

11. There are over a thousand chemicals in marijuana smoke.

Again, true but misleading. The 31 August 1990 issue of the magazine *Science* notes that of the over 800 volatile chemicals present in roasted *coffee*, only 21 have actually been tested on animals and 16 of these cause cancer in rodents. Yet, coffee remains legal and is generally considered fairly safe.

12. No one has ever died of a marijuana overdose.

This is true. It was put in to see if you are paying attention. Animal tests have revealed that extremely high doses of cannabinoids are needed to have lethal effect. This has led scientists to conclude that the ratio of the amount of cannabinoids necessary to get a person intoxicated (i.e., stoned) relative to the amount necessary to kill them is 1 to 40,000. In other words, to overdose, you would have to consume 40,000 times as much marijuana as you needed to get stoned. In contrast, the ratio for alcohol varies between 1 to 4 and 1 to 10. It is easy to see how upwards of 5000 people die from alcohol overdoses every year and no one *ever* dies of marijuana overdoses.

Sources

1. *Marijuana and Health,* Institute of Medicine, National Academy of Sciences, 1982. Note: the Committee on Substance Abuse and Habitual Behavior of the *Marijuana and Health* study had its part of the final

report suppressed when it reviewed the evidence and recommended that possession of small amounts of marijuana should no longer be a crime (*Time* magazine, July 19, 1982). The two *JAMA* studies are: Co, B.T., Goodwin, D.W., Gado, M., Mikhael, M., and Hill, S.Y.: "Absence of cerebral atrophy in chronic cannabis users", *JAMA,* 237:1229–1230, 1977; and, Kuehnle, J., Mendelson, J.H., Davis, K.R., and New, P.F.J.: "Computed tomographic examination of heavy marijuana smokers", *JAMA,* 237:1231–1232, 1977.

2. See *Marijuana and Health,* ibid., for information on this research. See also, *Marijuana Reconsidered* (1978) by Dr. Lester Grinspoon.

3. The Dutch experience is written up in "The Economics of Legalizing Drugs", by Richard J. Dennis, *The Atlantic Monthly,* vol. 266, no. 5, Nov. 1990, p. 130. See "A Comparison of Marijuana Users and Non-users" by Norman Zinberg and Andrew Weil (1971) for the negative correlation between use of marijuana and use of alcohol. The 1993 Rand Corporation study is "The Effect of Marijuana Decriminalization on Hospital Emergency Room Episodes: 1975–1978" by Karyn E. Model.

4. See a review of studies and their methodology in "Marijuana and Immunity", *Journal of Psychoactive Drugs,* vol. 20(1), Jan.–Mar. 1988.

5. The 90% figure comes from *Health Consequences of Smoking: Nicotine Addiction, Surgeon General's Report, 1988. In Health* magazine in an article entitled, "Hooked, Not Hooked" by Deborah Franklin (pp. 39–52), compares the addictives of various drugs and ranks marijuana below coffeine. For current information on cannabis drinks see *Working Men and Ganja: Marijuana Use in Rural Jamaica* by M.C. Dreher, Institute for the Study of Human Issues, 1982, ISBN 0-89727-025-8. For information on cannabis and actual cancer risk, see *Marijuana and Health,* ibid.

6. For a survey of studies relating to cannabis and highway accidents see "Marijuana, Driving and Accident Safety", by Dale Gieringer, *Journal of Psychoactive Drugs,* ibid. The effect of decriminalization on highway accidents is analyzed in "Do Youths Substitute Alcohol and Marijuana? Some Econometric Evidence" by Frank J. Chaloupka and Adit Laixuthai, Nov. 1992, University of Illinois at Chicago.

7. For information about the Partnership ad, see Jack Herer's book, *The Emperor Wears No Clothes,* 1990, p. 74. See also "Hard Sell in the Drug War", *The Nation,* March 9, 1992, by Cynthia Cotts, which reveals that the Partnership receives a large percentage of its advertizing budget from alcohol, tobacco, and pharmaceutical companies and is thus disposed toward exaggerating the risks of marijuana while downplaying the risks of legal drugs. For information on memory and the alpha brainwave enhancement effect, see "Marijuana, Memory, and Perception", by R.L. Dornbush, M.D., M. Fink, M.D., and A.M. Freedman, M.D., presented at the 124th annual meeting of the American Psychiatric Association, May 3–7, 1971.

8. See "Cannabis 1988, Old Drug New Dangers, The Potency Question" by Tod H Mikuriya, M.D. and Michael Aldrich, Ph.D., *Journal of Psychoactive Drugs,* ibid.

9. See *Marijuana and Health,* ibid. Also see "Marijuana, Memory, and Perception", ibid.

10. The fat solubility of cannabinoids and certain vitamins is well known. See *Marijuana and Health,* ibid. For some information on vitamin A, see "The A Team" in *Scientific American,* vol. 264, no. 2, February 1991, p. 16.

11. See "Too Many Rodent Carcinogens: Mitogenesis Increases Mutagenesis", Bruce N. Ames and Lois Swirsky Gold, *Science,* vol. 249, 31 August 1990, p. 971.

12. Cannabis and alcohol toxicity is compared in *Marijuana Reconsidered,* ibid., p. 227. Yearly alcohol overdoses was taken from "Drug Prohibition in the United States: Costs, Consequences, and Alternatives" by Ethan A. Nadelmann, *Science,* vol. 245, 1 September 1989, p. 943.

Marijuana's Addictive Effects

Ingrid Wickelgren

Research suggests that marijuana affects the brain in ways similar to addictive drugs such as heroin, reports Ingrid Wickelgren in the following selection. For instance, the author states, the same chemical produced during opiate withdrawal is released during withdrawal from marijuana. She notes that marijuana use triggers a surge of a pleasure-inducing chemical called dopamine, which is also released during heroin use, leading to dependence on the drug. According to the author, these similarities between marijuana and other addictive drugs may provide a biological basis for the controversial gateway theory, which hypothesizes that marijuana leads to the use of harder drugs such as heroin. Wickelgren writes frequently on issues related to molecular biology and neuroscience. She is a contributing correspondent for *Science* and a contributor to periodicals such as *Popular Science*, *Health Business Week*, and the *New York Times*.

For decades, policy-makers have debated whether to legalize marijuana. Compared to drugs such as heroin and cocaine, many people—scientists and teenagers alike—consider marijuana a relatively benign substance. Indeed, there was little evidence to indicate that it is addictive the way those drugs are. But now, two studies demonstrate disturbing similarities between marijuana's effects on the brain and those produced by highly addictive drugs such as cocaine, heroin, alcohol, and nicotine.

Researching Marijuana Addiction

In one study, a team of researchers from the Scripps Research Institute in La Jolla, California, and Complutense University of Madrid in Spain trace the symptoms of emotional stress caused by marijuana withdrawal to the same brain chemical, a peptide called corticotropin-releasing factor (CRF), that has already been linked to anxiety and stress during opiate, alcohol, and cocaine withdrawal. In the other study, Gaetano Di Chiara of the University of Cagliari in Italy and his colleagues report that the active ingredient in marijuana—a cannabinoid known as THC—results in the same key biochemical event that seems to reinforce dependence on other drugs, from nicotine to heroin: a release of dopamine in part of the brain's "reward" pathway.

Together, the two sets of experiments suggest that marijuana manipulates the brain's stress and reward systems in the same way as more potent drugs, to keep users coming back for more. "These two studies supply important evidence that marijuana acts on the same neural substrates and has the same effects as drugs already known to be highly addictive," says David Friedman, a neurobiologist at Bowman Gray School of Medicine in Winston-Salem, North Carolina. They also, he adds, "send a powerful message that should raise everyone's awareness about the dangers of marijuana use."

But the results may have a more hopeful message as well, because they may guide scientists in devising better strategies for treating marijuana dependence, for which some 100,000 people in the United States alone seek treatment each year. For instance, chemicals that block the effects of CRF or even relaxation exercises might ameliorate the miserable moods experienced by people in THC withdrawal. In addition, opiate antagonists like naloxone may, by dampening dopamine release, block the reinforcing properties of marijuana in people.

Scripps neuropharmacologists Friedbert Weiss and George Koob first began thinking that stress systems might be involved in drug dependence in the early 1990s, after noticing that withdrawal from many drugs produces an anxious, negative disposition that resembles an emotional response to stress. They reasoned that drug withdrawal might recruit the same brain structures and chemicals that are involved in the stress response. Because Koob's team had associated emotional stress with the release of CRF in a brain structure called the amygdala, they thought that drug withdrawal might also trigger CRF release.

Beginning in 1992, the Scripps researchers amassed evidence showing that this is indeed the case. First, Koob and his colleagues found that injecting chemicals that block CRF's effects into the amygdalas of alcohol-dependent rats reduces the anxiety-related symptoms, such as a reluctance to explore novel settings, that develop when the animals are taken off alcohol. Then in 1995, Weiss, Koob, and their colleagues showed that CRF levels quadruple in the amygdalas of rats during the peak of alcohol withdrawal.

After similar experiments demonstrated that elevated CRF underlies emotional withdrawal from opiates and cocaine, Weiss, Koob, and M. Rocío Carrera of Scripps, along with two visiting Spanish scientists, Fernando Rodríguez de Fonseca and Miguel Navarro, set out to investigate whether CRF might mediate the stressful malaise that some long-term marijuana users experience after quitting.

The researchers injected a synthetic cannabinoid into more than 50 rats once a day for 2 weeks to mimic the effects of heavy, long-term marijuana use in humans. Normally, marijuana withdrawal symptoms develop too gradually to be recognized easily in rats, because the body eliminates THC very slowly. But the researchers were able to produce a dramatic withdrawal syndrome lasting 80 minutes by injecting the rats with a newly developed drug that counteracts THC. The drug does this by binding to the receptor through which cannabinoids exert their effects.

The group found that the cannabinoid antagonist greatly increased the rats' anxiety, as measured in a standard behavioral test, and exaggerated such signs of stress as compulsive grooming and teeth chattering during withdrawal. What's more, when the scientists measured CRF levels in the rats' amygdalas, they found that rats in withdrawal had two to three times more CRF than controls not given the antagonist, and that the increase paralleled the apparent anxiety and stress levels of the rats.

The results, experts say, provide the first neurochemical basis for a marijuana withdrawal syndrome, and one with a strong emotional component that is shared by other abused drugs. "The work suggests that the CRF system may be a part of a common experience in withdrawal—that is, anxiety," says Alan Leshner, director of the National Institute on Drug Abuse. A desire to avoid this and other negative emotions, Weiss suggests, may prompt a vicious cycle leading to dependence.

The Brain's Reward System
But withdrawal is just one component of addiction. Addictive drugs also have immediate rewarding, or reinforcing, effects that keep people and animals coming back for more. The drugs produce these effects, scientists believe, by hijacking the brain's so-called reward system. A key event in the reward pathway is the release of dopamine by a small cluster of neurons in a brain region called the nucleus accumbens. Researchers think the dopamine release normally serves to reinforce behaviors that lead to biologically important rewards, such as food or sex. Addictive drugs are thought to lead to compulsive behavior because they unleash a dopamine surge of their own.

But no one had been able to show convincingly that marijuana could induce that telltale dopamine rush, until Di Chiara and his colleagues put THC to the test. When the Cagliari team infused the cannabinoid into a small group of rats and measured dopamine levels in the nucleus accumbens, they found that the levels jumped as much as twofold over those in the accumbens of control rats infused with an inactive cannabinoid. The magnitude of the surge was similar to what the researchers saw when they gave heroin to another set of rats.

Further work confirmed that cannabinoids, rather than other factors such as the stress of being handled by the experimenters, were responsible for the dopamine release. For example, the researchers observed no dopamine increase in animals who were given a receptor blocker before the THC.

Priming the Brain

Then Di Chiara and his colleagues found an additional parallel between THC and heroin. They showed that naloxone, a drug that blocks brain receptors for heroin and other opiates, prevents THC from raising dopamine levels, just as it does with heroin. This indicates that both marijuana and heroin boost dopamine by activating opiate receptors. Marijuana, however, presumably does so indirectly, by causing the release of an endogenous opiate: a heroinlike compound made in the brain. "Marijuana may provide one way of activating the endogenous opiate system," explains Di Chiara.

Di Chiara speculates that this overlap in the effects of THC and opiates on the reward pathway may provide a biological basis for the controversial "gateway hypothesis," in which smoking marijuana is thought to cause some people to abuse harder drugs. Marijuana, Di Chiara suggests, may prime the brain to seek substances like heroin that act in a similar way. Koob and Weiss add that the stress and anxiety brought on by marijuana withdrawal might also nudge a user toward harder drugs.

More work will be needed to confirm these ideas, as well as to find out exactly how marijuana influences the stress and reward systems. For instance, nobody knows how THC interacts with neurons in the amygdala to alter the release of CRF. Nor do scientists understand the molecular steps by which THC triggers the dopamine release in the nucleus accumbens.

But despite these uncertainties, both papers should help revise the popular perception of pot as a relatively—although not completely—safe substance to something substantially more sinister. "I would be satisfied if, following all this evidence, people would no longer consider THC a 'soft' drug," says Di Chiara. "I'm not saying it's as dangerous as heroin, but I'm hoping people will approach marijuana far more cautiously than they have before."

Marijuana Is Not a Gateway Drug

John P. Morgan and Lynn Zimmer

John P. Morgan is a physician and a professor of pharmacology at the City University of New York's medical school. Lynn Zimmer is an associate professor of sociology at Queens College, City University of New York. They are the authors of *Marijuana Myths, Marijuana Facts: A Review of the Scientific Evidence*. In the following article, Morgan and Zimmer examine the hypothesis that marijuana serves as a "gateway" to the use of more dangerous drugs. This theory is a myth employed by anti-drug organizations, they contend. According to the authors, nearly seventy million Americans who have tried marijuana have not progressed to harder drugs. In fact, they write, marijuana use decreased throughout the 1980s, while cocaine use was on the rise. These divergent patterns suggest that there is no causal link between marijuana and cocaine use, the authors argue.

The Partnership for a Drug-Free America, in cooperation with the National Institute on Drug Abuse (NIDA) and the White House Office of Drug Control Policy, recently announced a new anti-drug campaign that specifically targets marijuana. Instead of featuring horror tales of marijuana-induced insanity, violence and birth defects, this campaign is built upon the premise that reducing marijuana use is a practical strategy for reducing the use of more dangerous drugs.

Examining the Statistics

The primary basis for this "gateway hypothesis" is a recent report by the center on Addiction and Substance Abuse (CASA), claiming that marijuana users are 85 times more likely than non-marijuana users to try cocaine. This figure, using data from NIDA's 1991 National Household Survey on Drug Abuse, is close to being meaningless. It was calculated by dividing the proportion of marijuana users who have ever used cocaine (17%) by the proportion of cocaine users who have never used marijuana (.2%). The high risk-factor obtained is a product not of the fact that so many marijuana users use cocaine but that so

Reprinted, with permission, from "The Myth of Marijuana's Gateway Effect," by John P. Morgan and Lynn Zimmer, www.druglibrary.org/schaffer/LIBRARY/mjgate.html.

many cocaine users used marijuana previously.

It is hardly a revelation that people who use one of the least popular drugs are likely to use the more popular ones—not only marijuana, but also alcohol and tobacco cigarettes. The obvious statistic not publicized by CASA is that most marijuana users—83 percent—never use cocaine. Indeed, for the nearly 70 million Americans who have tried marijuana, it is clearly a "terminus" rather than a "gateway" drug.

During the last few years, after a decade of decline, there has been a slight increase in marijuana use, particularly among youth. In 1994, 38 percent of high school seniors reported having ever tried the drug, compared to about 35 percent in 1993 and 33 percent in 1992. This increase does not constitute a crisis. No one knows whether marijuana use-rates will continue to rise. But even if they do, it will not necessarily lead to increased use of cocaine.

Since the 1970s, when NIDA first began gathering data, rates of marijuana and cocaine use have displayed divergent patterns. Marijuana prevalence increased throughout the 1970s, peaking in 1979, when about 60 percent of high school seniors reported having used it at least once. During the 1980s, cocaine use increased while marijuana use was declining. Since 1991, when data for the CASA analysis were gathered, marijuana use-rates have increased while cocaine use-rates have remained fairly steady.

The ever-changing nature of the statistical relationship between use-rate for marijuana and cocaine indicates the absence of a causal link between the use of these two drugs. Therefore, even if the proposed Partnership campaign were to be effective in reducing marijuana use it would not guarantee a proportional reduction in the number of people who use cocaine. To the extent anti-drug campaigns are effective, they seem to be most effective in deterring those people who would have been fairly low-level users. There is no reason to believe that anti-marijuana messages of any sort would deter many of those marijuana users—currently 17 percent of the total—who also develop an interest in cocaine.

Nor is there reason to believe that the Partnership's new campaign will actually reduce the overall number of marijuana users. For a decade now, American youth have been subjected to an unparalleled assault of anti-drug messages. They have seen hundreds of Partnership advertisements, on television and in the print media. They have been urged to "just say no" by rock stars, sports heroes, presidents and first ladies. They have been exposed to anti-drug educational programs in the schools. Yet this is the same generation of young people that recently began increasing its use of marijuana. It seems unlikely that many of them will be deterred by hyperbolic claims of marijuana's gateway effect, particularly when it contradicts the reality of drug use they see around them.

If the creators of American drug policy are truly interested in reducing the risk of marijuana users using other drugs, they should take a closer look at Holland, where drug policy since the 1970s has been guided by a commitment to diminishing any potential gateway effect. Wanting to keep young marijuana users away from cocaine and other "hard drugs," the Dutch decided to separate the retail markets by allowing anyone 18 years of age or older to purchase marijuana openly in government-controlled "coffee shops" which strictly prohibit the use and sale of other drugs.

Despite easy availability, marijuana prevalence among 12 to 18 year olds in Holland is only 13.6 percent—well below the 38 percent use-rate for American high school seniors. More Dutch teenagers use marijuana now than in the past; indeed, lifetime prevalence increased nearly three-fold between 1984 and 1992, from 4.8 to 13.6 percent. However, Dutch officials consider their policy a success because the increase in marijuana use has not been accompanied by an increase in the use of other drugs. For the last decade, the rate of cocaine use among Dutch youth has remained stable, with about .3 percent of 12–18 year olds reporting having used it in the past month.

In the United States, the claim that marijuana acts as a gateway to the use of other drugs serves mainly as a rhetorical tool for frightening Americans into believing that winning the war against heroin and cocaine requires waging a battle against the casual use of marijuana. Not only is the claim intellectually indefensible, but the battle is wasteful of resources and fated to failure.

Marijuana Use Impairs Driving

Judy Monroe

In the following selection, Judy Monroe explores the hazards of driving while using marijuana. She explains that marijuana use impairs the skills needed for safe driving: It slows reaction time, causes drowsiness and forgetfulness, adversely affects vision, and increases the likelihood of making mistakes while driving. Drivers who use marijuana are easily distracted by sights and sounds rather than remaining focused on their driving, Monroe reports. In particular, the author observes, teenagers who drive while high on marijuana significantly increase their chances of causing an accident. Monroe is a staff writer for *Current Health 2*.

"At age 18, I was living with my sister and her family. I didn't have much privacy there, so my friends and I got high on pot [marijuana] in our cars a lot." Sunnie R. paused.

"I remember the first time I got high. It was the night of the January [17, 1994,] earthquake [in Northridge, California]. My girlfriend was driving along the 405 freeway in California, and I was in the backseat. My friends were passing around a bong—it's like a waterpipe that concentrates a lot of marijuana smoke. The first time I tried it, the smoke made me cough and burned my throat and lungs. After another hit, I didn't care about the pain, as I got high."

Sunnie began to smoke pot regularly, with friends or by herself. "As a result of using pot, I got absentminded. I constantly forgot to turn off my car lights and would wear down the battery. Or I'd forget to change the oil and almost burned out the engine several times. Expensive car repairs piled up.

"One time when I was high, I really messed up my sister's car. Pot slows down your motor reflexes, so it's hard to operate a car. I kept trying to park her car and got too close to a wall and ruined the outside with scratches and dings all over. She was so mad at me.

"Pot also impairs your ability to make good judgment calls. The drug convinces you that you're making good choices. Instead, I'd do such stupid things. I'd drive around by myself in very unsafe areas and do dumb things like forgetting where I was. I'd mistake people for shadows and nearly hit them.

"One night, my car transmission went out in a bad area. I sat there for two hours, scared to flag down the police because if they realized I was high, I could go to jail. I finally fell asleep, and when I woke up the next morning, someone had stolen my hubcaps, but I was OK. My brother-in-law was furious when he came and got me."

Her family called a meeting the next day and told Sunnie she had to get help. "By this time, I was in bad shape. Marijuana had taken away my goals, dreams, and desires. I was living minute-to-minute," Sunnie says.

Drugs and Driving Do Not Mix

Studies have shown that marijuana plays a role in crashes. And when users combine marijuana with alcohol, the hazards of driving can be more severe than with either drug alone.

Marijuana affects drivers' ability to focus, visually follow, and pay attention to what is going on around their vehicle. Drivers who are high become disoriented. This increases the chances of missing turning cars or cars entering a highway from a ramp. Marijuana decreases peripheral vision and can affect depth perception, so drivers may miss seeing cars or pedestrians off to the side. Because distances seem longer and objects may seem larger, drivers who are high may run into vehicles stopped at lights.

According to the National Institute on Drug Abuse, one study of patients in a hospital's shock-trauma unit who had been in traffic accidents found that 15 percent had been smoking marijuana; 17 percent had both alcohol and THC (delta-9-tetrahydrocannabinol, the main active chemical in marijuana) in their blood.

Effects on the Body

Marijuana affects people differently. Some may feel nothing when they first try it. Others may feel high or intoxicated, as if they're drunk. Because they're so relaxed and drowsy, they may fall asleep behind the wheel.

Users often become engrossed with ordinary sights, sounds, or tastes, and minor events may seem extremely interesting or funny. This is bad news for drivers. Users don't focus on driving and instead may get wrapped up in music on the radio, for example. While high, time seems to pass slowly, so minutes seem like hours. Users tend to have poor reaction times while driving, misjudging how long it takes to slow down or to stop the car.

Bad reactions can occur, especially with high doses of THC or if marijuana is mixed with other drugs such as cocaine. As Sunnie learned, "You never know what you're getting when you buy pot. Sometimes it's laced with cocaine, LSD, or speed."

Marijuana reacts quickly in the body. Within a few minutes, users develop dry mouth, rapid heartbeat, some loss of coordination, a poor sense of balance, and decreased reaction time. Blood vessels in the eye expand, making eyes look red. For some people, marijuana raises blood pressure.

THC can last a long time in the body because body fat absorbs THC. This means that urine testing can detect THC several days after a smoking session. In heavy, chronic users, the chemical can be detected for weeks or months, even if a person has stopped using marijuana.

When Sunnie used marijuana, she had trouble with thinking and problem-solving. These effects are typical of marijuana users.

Marijuana affects short-term memory—that is, memory of recent events. THC disrupts the nerve cells in the part of the brain where memories are formed. In turn, this makes it hard to learn while high.

When high, the person is more likely to make mistakes. The mistakes could be embarrassing or even cause a car crash. And like Sunnie, when people use marijuana a lot, they may lose energy and interest in school, work, family, and life.

Once her family forced Sunnie to admit she was addicted to marijuana, she got help. With a lot of work, Sunnie stopped using marijuana. "I've been sober since April 1994." Now 21, Sunnie is rebuilding her life.

THE TRUTH BEHIND PROPAGANDA ABOUT MARIJUANA'S ADVERSE EFFECTS

Jacob Sullum

The claims made about the negative effects of marijuana are similar to those concerning tobacco at the start of the twentieth century, argues Jacob Sullum in the following selection. Sullum explains that opponents of tobacco blamed smoking for increases in crime, lower productivity rates, and the delinquency of America's youth. Marijuana's opponents make the same claims today, the author contends. For example, opponents of tobacco maintained that cigarette smoking dulled the mind, leading many businesses to refuse to hire smokers. Likewise, Sullum points out, in 1991, the Partnership for a Drug-Free America warned that U.S. businesses were losing money because of marijuana use, prompting many companies to begin testing employees for drugs. Such propaganda appeals to societal fears while failing to confront the truth about marijuana's effects, he asserts. Sullum is a senior editor for *Reason*, a libertarian opinion magazine, and author of *For Your Own Good: The Anti-Smoking Crusade and the Tyranny of Public Health*.

It makes you stupid. It turns teenagers into ne'er-do-wells and juvenile delinquents. It ruins academic performance, stifles ambition, and impairs efficiency at work. It leads to the use of other drugs. Today it's marijuana. Eighty years ago, it was tobacco, especially in the form of cigarettes.

"No boy or man can expect to succeed in this world to a high position and continue the use of cigarettes," Philadelphia Athletics Manager Connie Mack wrote in 1913. Biologist David Starr Jordan, the first president of Stanford University, concurred. "The boy who smokes cigarettes need not be anxious about his future," he said. "He has none."

In 1914 the industrialist Henry Ford published *The Case Against the*

Little White Slaver, which included condemnations of cigarettes from entrepreneurs, educators, community leaders, and athletes. Thomas Edison, who contributed to Ford's booklet, was simply repeating a widely accepted notion when he observed that cigarette smoke "has a violent action on the nerve centers, producing degeneration of the cells of the brain, which is quite rapid among boys. Unlike most narcotics this degeneration is permanent and uncontrollable."

Examining Propaganda Campaigns

The anti-tobacco propaganda of this period, when marijuana was still legal but cigarettes were banned in more than a dozen states, shares some prominent themes with contemporary anti-pot propaganda. Opponents of tobacco depicted cigarettes as a foreign threat to the youth of America, sapping their energy and intelligence. They described the effects of cigarettes in terms that would later be associated with the "amotivational syndrome" supposedly caused by marijuana. They claimed that smoking led to crime, brain damage, lower productivity, and narcotic addiction. In response, they urged children to make pledges of abstinence.

These similarities are especially striking because of the marked pharmacological differences between tobacco and marijuana. The parallels suggest that responses to drug use have less to do with the inherent properties of the substance than with perennial fears that are projected onto the chemical menace of the day.

This is not to say that tobacco and marijuana are harmless. The anti-cigarette movement is far more influential today than it was in 1914, mainly because of scientific evidence that has emerged since then concerning the long-term health consequences of smoking. But today's anti-smoking activists worry about lung cancer, heart disease, and emphysema, not laziness, crime, and brain damage. When they claim that smoking hurts productivity, they are thinking of the habit's effect on physical health, not its impact on ambition or intellect. Despite the continuing controversy over smoking, the concerns about mental decay and moral corruption voiced by opponents of cigarettes early in the twentieth century seem quaint and fanciful today.

When it comes to marijuana, however, those charges still ring true with many Americans. There is some basis, after all, for pothead stereotypes. People who are under the influence of marijuana most of the time, like people who are drunk most of the time, may not get good grades in school or promotions at work. But that does not mean that occasional marijuana use renders people incapable of academic or professional success, any more than an occasional drink does. The staunchest opponents of marijuana invest the drug with the power to permanently transform people, ruining their potential and turning them against society. Before we accept that notion, it's worth reflecting on the fact that people once said much the same thing about cigarettes.

Reactions to Marijuana Use

Historical perspective is especially important in light of recent trends. According to government-sponsored surveys, teenage marijuana use has been rising since 1992, following a 13-year decline. In the National Household Survey, the share of 12-to-17-year-olds reporting past-month use of marijuana rose from 4 percent in 1992 to 6 percent in 1994. In the Monitoring the Future Survey, the share of high school seniors who said they had used marijuana in the previous year rose from 21.9 percent in 1992 to 34.7 percent in 1995. These figures are still well below the peak levels seen in 1979 (16.8 percent and 50.8 percent, respectively), but the increases have aroused concern among parents and educators.

Citing the survey data, drug warriors such as Sen. Orrin Hatch (R-Utah) have criticized the Clinton administration for not doing enough to suppress drug use and have called for greater emphasis on interdiction and enforcement. But the government is already arresting more people for marijuana possession than ever before, suggesting that another crackdown may not be effective. Furthermore, alcohol and tobacco use are also rising among teenagers, something that President Bill Clinton's lack of enthusiasm for the war on drugs can hardly explain. Given the emotional resonance of pot-smoking kids, however, there is a real danger that Clinton or a Republican successor will take Hatch's advice, pushing the pendulum of drug policy back toward the hysteria of the late 1980s. In this context, the parallels between current fears about marijuana and earlier fears about tobacco are instructive. They do not demonstrate that worries about pot are entirely illusory, but they suggest that we should be wary of overreaction.

Although tobacco had been widely used by Americans since colonial times, cigarettes did not catch on until after production was mechanized in the 1880s. Per capita consumption of cigarettes rose nearly a hundredfold between 1870 and 1890, from less than one to more than 35. In 1900 chewing tobacco, cigars, and pipes were still more popular, but by 1910 cigarettes had become the leading tobacco product in the United States. Per capita consumption skyrocketed from 85 that year to nearly 1,000 in 1930.

The rise of the cigarette caused alarm not only among diehard opponents of tobacco but also among pipe and cigar smokers (such as Edison), who perceived the new product as qualitatively different. Critics believed (rightly) that cigarettes were more dangerous to health because the smoke was typically inhaled. They also worried that boys and women would be attracted by the product's milder smoke and low price. "The cigarette is designed for boys and women," *The New York Times* declared in 1884. "The decadence of Spain began when the Spaniards adopted cigarettes, and if this pernicious practice obtains among adult Americans the ruin of the Republic is close at hand."

A Comparison of the Propaganda

At first the anti-cigarette campaign, which had close ties to the temperance movement, focused on restricting children's access. By 1890, 26 states had passed laws forbidding cigarette sales to minors, but many children continued to smoke. Led by Lucy Page Gaston, a former teacher from Illinois whose career as a social reformer began in the Women's Christian Temperance Union, the anti-cigarette crusaders next insisted that complete prohibition was necessary to protect the youth of America. Between 1893 and 1921, 14 states and one territory (Oklahoma) enacted laws banning the sale of cigarettes, and in some cases possession as well. Such laws were supported by the cigar industry, which saw its business slipping away to a new competitor.

Upholding Tennessee's ban in 1898, the state Supreme Court declared that cigarettes "are wholly noxious and deleterious to health. Their use is always harmful; never beneficial. They possess no virtue, but are inherently bad, bad only. They find no true commendation for merit or usefulness in any sphere. On the contrary, they are widely condemned as pernicious altogether. Beyond any question, their every tendency is toward the impairment of physical health and mental vigor."

In contrast to contemporary anti-smoking activists, who talk almost exclusively about the habit's effect on the body, turn-of-the-century critics were just as concerned about its impact on the mind. In the 1904 edition of *Our Bodies and How We Live*, an elementary school textbook, Dr. Albert F. Blaisdell warned: "The cells of the brain may become poisoned from tobacco. The ideas may lack clearness of outline. The will power may be weakened, and it may be an effort to do the routine duties of life. . . . The memory may also be impaired."

Blaisdell also reported that "the honors of the great schools, academies, and colleges are very largely taken by the abstainers from tobacco. . . . The reason for this is plain. The mind of the habitual user of tobacco is apt to lose its capacity for study or successful effort. This is especially true of boys and young men. The growth and development of the brain having been once retarded, the youthful user of tobacco has established a permanent drawback which may hamper him all his life. The keenness of his mental perception may be dulled and his ability to seize and hold an abstract thought may be impaired."

In the 1908 textbook *The Human Body and Health*, biologist Alvin Davison agreed that tobacco "prevents the brain cells from developing to their full extent and results in a slow and dull mind." He added, "At Harvard University during fifty years no habitual user of tobacco ever graduated at the head of his class."

Reinforcing the Stereotypes

The dull, listless underachievers described by Blaisdell, Davison, and other tobacco opponents resemble contemporary portrayals of marijuana users. In 1989 William Bennett, then director of the Office of

National Drug Control Policy, explained how smoking pot affects young people: "It means they don't study. It causes what is called 'amotivational syndrome' where they are just not motivated to get up and go to work."

The Partnership for a Drug-Free America, which is supported partly by donations from tobacco companies, has helped reinforce this stereotype. One of the Partnership's television spots shows two young men smoking marijuana, one watching TV, the other ridiculing warnings about the dangers of pot: "We've been smoking for 15 years, and nothing has ever happened to me." Then we hear the voice of his mother asking him if he's looked for a job today. "Marijuana can make nothing happen to you, too," the announcer says.

Another Partnership commercial shows a stoned teenager turning down invitations from friends to play baseball, go skate-boarding, or listen to music. "You always thought marijuana would take you places," the announcer says. "So how come you're going nowhere?" The most notorious anti-pot ad from the Partnership purported to contrast a normal EEG reading with the EEG reading of a marijuana smoker. It was later revealed that the second display actually showed the brain waves of someone asleep or in a coma. Another spot, "No Brainer," compared the effects of smoking marijuana to the effects of being repeatedly hit in the head by a professional boxer.

The tricks of anti-pot propaganda are usually more subtle, however. A common approach is to cite the immediate effects of smoking marijuana without noting that they disappear when the drug wears off. In a joint statement that accompanied the release of a 1995 report called *Legalization: Panacea or Pandora's Box* (you can guess which side they came down on), Bennett and Joseph Califano, the former Health, Education, and Welfare secretary who heads the Center on Addiction and Substance Abuse, said that "marijuana use . . . savages short-term memory, sharply curtails ability to concentrate and diminishes motor functions."

A pamphlet from DARE (Drug Abuse Resistance Education) declares, "Young people who smoke marijuana heavily over long periods of time can become dull, slow-moving, and inattentive. These 'burned-out' users are sometimes so unaware of their surroundings that they do not respond when friends speak to them, and they do not realize they have a problem." In the 1985 book *Marijuana Alert*, Peggy Mann suggested that diminished mental capacity is a persistent trait of pot smokers, intoxicated or not.

Promoters of this idea will be photocopying a study that appeared in the February 21, 1996, *Journal of the American Medical Association*. The researchers found that, after abstaining for at least 19 hours, heavy pot smokers (who used marijuana daily or almost daily) performed slightly worse on tests of learning and attentiveness than occasional pot smokers did. (The two groups scored about the same on basic memory tests.) Since the heavy users were more likely to have smoked marijuana recently, the results may indicate a "hangover" effect.

The lead researcher, Harvard psychiatrist Harrison G. Pope Jr., told *Harvard Magazine* that, among the light smokers, "total lifetime consumption did *not* predict results on the cognitive tests. . . . My bet is that there really is a residual effect caused by drug residue." Another possibility is that people who are inclined to smoke pot heavily are, on average, somewhat less attentive than other people to begin with. A third possibility is that the heavy smokers were used to functioning under the influences of marijuana and were distracted by its absence. Although this study does not demonstrate permanent impairment (or negative effects from occasional use), anti-pot propagandists will probably use it to keep alive the notion that marijuana causes brain damage.

The Fears of Employers

Employers are not eager to hire dim-witted layabouts, whatever they're smoking. "The time is already at hand when smokers will be barred out of positions which demand quick thought and action," wrote Charles B. Towns, operator of a New York drug and alcohol hospital, in 1912. Thomas Edison declared, "I employ no person who smokes cigarettes." With Edison and Henry Ford leading the way, many prominent businessmen adopted the same policy during the first two decades of the twentieth century. Hundreds of large companies, including Montgomery Ward and Sears Roebuck, refused to hire smokers.

Similarly, in the 1980s and '90s employers have become increasingly concerned about the impact of marijuana and other illegal drugs on productivity. Many companies now require job applicants to undergo urine tests, a policy encouraged by hyperbolic claims about the costs of drug use. "Last year alone," asserted a series of Partnership for a Drug-Free America ads in 1991, "America's businesses lost more than $60 billion to drugs. So this year, most of the Fortune 500 will be administering drug tests." The $60 billion figure, which was also cited by President George Bush and widely reported in the news media, included an estimate of "reduced productivity due to daily marijuana use." The estimate came from a 1982 study that found adults who had smoked marijuana for at least 20 out of 30 days (at any point in their lives) had lower household incomes, on average, than adults who hadn't. The researchers simply assumed that the difference was due to the influence of marijuana.

Creating a Link to Crime

In addition to their alleged effects on motivation, intellectual performance, and productivity, both tobacco and marijuana have been tied to crime. "Recent careful investigations by many persons," Davison reported in his 1908 book, *The Human Body and Health*, "show that cigarette smoking not only clouds the intellect, but tends to make criminals of boys. Dr. Hutchison, of the Kansas State Reformatory, says: 'Using cigarettes is the cause of the downfall of more of the inmates of this institution than all other vicious habits combined.' Of 4117 boys received into the Illinois State Reformatory, 4000 were in the habit of using tobacco, and over 3000 were cigarette smokers." In 1904 Charles B. Hubbell recalled that during his service as president of New York City's Board of Education, "it was found that nearly all of the incorrigible truants were cigaret fiends." He added that "the Police Magistrates of this and other cities have stated again and again that the majority of juvenile delinquents appearing before them are cigaret fiends whose moral nature has been warped or destroyed through the instrumentality of this vice."

While most of the critics who blamed cigarettes for crime implied that the effect was pharmacological, Henry Ford had a somewhat more sophisticated theory. "If you will study the history of almost any criminal you will find that he is an inveterate cigarette smoker," he said. "Boys, through cigarettes, train with bad company. They go with other smokers to the pool rooms and saloons. The cigarette drags them down."

Although drug warriors nowadays rarely claim that marijuana causes crime, that charge played an important role in building support for state and federal prohibition in the 1920s and '30s. A 1938 book, *Marijuana, America's New Drug Problem*, quoted an account by New Orleans Public Safety Commissioner Frank Gomila of a "crime wave" in the late '20s: "Youngsters known to be 'muggle-heads' fortified themselves with the narcotic and proceeded to shoot down police, bank clerks and casual bystanders. Mr. Eugene Stanley, at that time District Attorney, declared that many of the crimes in New Orleans and the south were thus committed by criminals who relied on the drug to give them false courage and freedom from restraint. Dr. George Roeling, Coroner, reported that of 450 prisoners investigated, 125 were confirmed users of marihuana. Mr. W.B. Graham, State Narcotic Officer, declared in 1936 that 60 percent of the crimes committed in New Orleans were by marihuana users."

Harry J. Anslinger, head of the Federal Bureau of Narcotics from 1932 to 1970, promoted the notion that marijuana causes violence to generate support for a national ban. During the '30s lurid newspaper and magazine stories about marijuana murders—in one case, a Florida youth was said to have hacked his family to death with an ax while under the influence—helped create a climate of alarm.

Appealing to Parents' Fears

Tobacco and marijuana have also been charged with subtler effects on behavior. "The action of any narcotic is to break down the sense of moral responsibility," wrote Towns, the drug treatment entrepreneur, in 1912. "If a father finds that his boy is fibbing to him, is difficult to manage, or does not wish to work, he will generally find that the boy is smoking cigarettes. . . . The action of a narcotic produces a peculiar cunning and resource in concealment." Noting the rudeness of smokers who light up despite the complaints of bystanders, Towns concluded that "callous indifference to the rights of others" was another effect of the drug. In *Our Bodies and How We Live*, Blaisdell agreed that "the effect of tobacco on the moral nature often shows itself in a selfish disregard for the rights of others."

It seems that pot, too, fosters dishonesty and rudeness. "Among the psychological effects of heavy pot use cited by teachers and parents," *The New York Times Magazine* reported in 1980, "are a loss of interest in schoolwork, a tendency to lie without feelings of guilt ('She stared me straight in the face,' one mother said of her junior-high-school daughter, 'tears running down her cheeks, swearing she was telling the truth about something, and I knew she was lying') and a change in attitude toward the family. 'I realized,' said a woman of her 12-year-old, 'that right under our noses our happy, lovely little girl had turned into a sullen, alienated, unreasonable creature.'" As these accounts suggest, the symptoms of marijuana use, like the symptoms of tobacco use, are often hard to distinguish from the symptoms of adolescence.

A 1990 booklet produced by the U.S. Department of Education, *Growing Up Drug Free: A Parent's Guide to Prevention*, offered a list of warning signs: "Does your child seem withdrawn, depressed, tired, and careless about personal grooming? Has your child become hostile and uncooperative? Have your child's relationships with other family members deteriorated? Has your child dropped his old friends? Is your child no longer doing well in school—grades slipping, attendance irregular? Has your child lost interest in hobbies, sports, and other favorite activities? Have your child's eating or sleeping patterns changed? Positive answers to any of these questions can indicate alcohol or other drug use." On the other hand, the booklet conceded, "it is sometimes hard to know the difference between normal teenage behavior and behavior caused by drugs."

The Gateway Theory

Tobacco and marijuana have been condemned not only because of their inherent dangers but because they supposedly lead to the use of other drugs. The psychiatric pioneer Benjamin Rush offered an early version of the "gateway" or "stepping-stone" theory in 1798. Rush, who had already described the inexorable slide into habitual drunkenness among those who developed a taste for liquor, said chewing or smoking tobacco contributed to alcoholism by creating a peculiar kind of thirst: "This thirst cannot be allayed by water, for no sedative or even insipid liquor will be relished after the mouth and throat have been exposed to the stimulus of the smoke, or juice of Tobacco. A desire of course is excited for strong drinks, and these when taken between meals soon lead to intemperance and drunkenness." In 1912 Towns took the notion a step further, saying tobacco leads to alcohol, and alcohol leads to morphine.

The gateway theory is also the last resort of drug warriors who are frustrated by the lack of evidence that marijuana is a menace. In the 1984 book *Getting Tough on Gateway Drugs*, Robert DuPont estimated that "up to 50 percent of regular users of marijuana also use heroin." In its 1995 paper on drug legalization, Califano's Center on Addiction and Substance Abuse reported that "12 to 17 year olds who smoke marijuana are 85 times more likely to use cocaine than those who do not."

Formulations of this kind obscure two crucial points: First, most marijuana users never even try another illegal drug, let alone use it regularly. Second, it is not safe to conclude from the fact that marijuana users are *more likely* to use heroin or cocaine that marijuana use *results in* heroin or cocaine use. (It is probably also true that adults who wear jeans more than three days a week and people who ride motorcycles without a helmet are more likely to try heroin or cocaine.) In this case as in so many others, anti-drug polemicists tend to confuse correlation with causation.

Pledging to Abstain

Given the hazards thought to be associated with tobacco and marijuana use, the safest course would seem to be early intervention aimed at preventing youthful experimentation. Accordingly, opponents of both drugs have formulated abstinence pledges, a device borrowed from the temperance movement.

George Trask, a Massachusetts minister who founded the American Anti-Tobacco Society in 1850, visited schools around the country and urged young people to take the Band of Hope pledge: "I hereby solemnly promise to abstain from the use of all Intoxicating Liquors as a beverage; I also promise to abstain from the use of Tobacco in all forms, and all Profane Language." In the 1890s Lucy Page Gaston adopted a similar strategy, leading boys and girls in the Clean Life Pledge: "I hereby pledge myself with the help of God to abstain from all intoxicating liquors as a beverage and from the use of tobacco in any form."

In the 1980s First Lady Nancy Reagan, who adopted drug education as her pet cause, famously urged children to "Just Say No." Kids who joined the clubs sponsored by Just Say No International had to sign this statement: "I pledge to lead a drug-free life. I want to be healthy and happy. I will say no to harmful drugs. I will help my friends say no. I pledge to stand up for what I know is right."

These pledges may seem naïve and simplistic, but they reflect a perfectly understandable desire to protect children from danger and make sure they grow up right. Current fears about marijuana and other illegal drugs, like turn-of-the-century fears about cigarettes, express the sort of worries that reappear in every generation. Parents naturally want their children to be smart, to do well in school, to respect authority, and to become productive, responsible adults. The dull, lazy, rebellious, and possibly criminal teenager—the cigarette fiend or pothead—is every parent's nightmare. Adults who have no children of their own worry that other people's kids will become tomorrow's parasites or predators, bringing decline and disorder.

Despite all the alarm that drug scares seem to generate, projecting these fears onto physical objects can be reassuring: Just keep the kids away from tobacco or marijuana (or alcohol or LSD), we are implicitly told, and they will turn out OK. As symbols of all the things that might go wrong on the path from birth to maturity, drugs offer what every adult confronted by a troublesome teenager longs for: the illusion of control.

CHAPTER 2

SHOULD MARIJUANA BE LEGALIZED?

Contemporary Issues
Companion

The Debate over the Legalization of Marijuana: An Overview

Paul Van Slambrouck

Paul Van Slambrouck examines both sides of the controversy over legalizing marijuana in the following selection. Supporters of legalization, he explains, assert that marijuana is a harmless drug that should be available for both medical and recreational use. They also argue that the prosecution of recreational marijuana users has failed to keep the drug off the streets, he relates. On the other hand, the author reports, opponents of legalization contend that marijuana use can lead young people to experiment with harder drugs. Van Slambrouck points out that the federal government continues to oppose legalizing even medical marijuana in the concern that any loosening of drug laws will have harmful repercussions in society. Van Slambrouck is a staff writer for the *Christian Science Monitor*, an international newspaper.

In a year when Woodstock makes headlines and Austin Powers does well at the box office, another 1960s phenomenon is attempting its own comeback: legalization of marijuana.

Even as the courts, law enforcement, and the federal government continue to wrestle with growing acceptance of marijuana for medicinal purposes, advocates have begun the first serious campaign in decades to erase penalties for its recreational use.

Billboards are sprouting up across San Francisco, laced with some humor, but carrying the tagline: "Stop arresting responsible pot smokers."

"We decided it was time to try and move the marijuana debate beyond the medicinal issue," says Keith Stroup, founder of the Washington-based National Organization for the Reform of Marijuana Laws, which is behind the new campaign.

While San Francisco, with its liberal reputation, was chosen as the launch site for the campaign, it is likely to spread to Los Angeles and other major cities in the coming months, Mr. Stroup says. The goal, he says, is to "introduce the concept of responsible marijuana use" by adults.

Sending the Wrong Message?

Opponents worry about a nascent softening of marijuana laws in general, and object in particular to the ripple effect of this newest campaign.

"This message is dangerous because it tells teens that marijuana is a benign drug," says Joseph Califano, president of the National Center on Addiction and Substance Abuse at Columbia University in New York. In reality, marijuana is a gateway drug that can lead to use of cocaine and other harder drugs, according to the center.

While backers of the new campaign favor legalization, they're attempting as a first step revival of the decriminalization trend that took hold from the late 1960s through 1978.

During that decade, 11 states passed laws reducing penalties, generally to a fine, for the private use of small amounts of marijuana. The movement was broad and embraced states as dissimilar as Nebraska, North Carolina, New York, Mississippi, Oregon, and California.

Then in the 1980s, the nation's political environment changed dramatically, with soaring public angst over crime and the general direction of the nation's youth. By the 1990s, the war on drugs was under way and marijuana advocates had shifted their strategy to focus more narrowly on legalizing the drug for medicinal purposes.

Now marijuana proponents think the nation's mood is shifting once again and that, for a variety of reasons, sentiment favoring liberalization is building anew. The Marijuana Policy Project, a Washington group involved in the effort to permit medical marijuana, predicts that the number of states allowing such use will double from four currently to eight or so over the next 18 months. Maine will vote in November 1999 on a medical marijuana initiative, with other states to follow in 2000 with ballot initiatives or legislation.

Shift in Federal Research

While the Clinton administration [1993–2001] has been a staunch opponent of loosening marijuana laws, that line of opposition was breached early in 1999 when the Institute of Medicine ruled, after assessing a wide range of scientific studies, that marijuana can be effective as medicine.

The study, requested by the White House, ran counter to the administration's previous insistence that there was no evidence marijuana had any beneficial role in treating the ill.

The Institute of Medicine finding has prompted new guidelines for scientific research on a number of remaining issues related to medical marijuana. Proponents consider the move a major step forward after years when the government basically blocked additional inquiry.

Still, the federal government has not softened its position that federal law prohibiting marijuana trumps state laws allowing medicinal use.

Early in August 1999, federal prosecutors won their first case against someone growing marijuana since California passed its medicinal marijuana initiative in 1996. A federal judge in Sacramento, disallowing any consideration of the state's voter-approved law, sentenced B.E. Smith to 27 months in prison for growing 87 pot plants.

Stroup says people are "fed up with the notion that we need to send everyone to prison for minor drug offenses," particularly for activities sanctioned by states. In fact, legislation in Congress would allow states to set medicinal-use policies without federal interference.

Most polls show strong public support of medical marijuana use, but most people do not favor legalization. Positions on decriminalization, where recreational use is punished with fines rather than jail, are less clear and depend on how the questions are phrased.

Decriminalization advocates say "prohibition" is a policy failure. The costs of funneling small-time marijuana users through the criminal courts far outweigh any discernible gains, they argue, particularly when penalties have not deterred the flood of marijuana on the streets. About 695,000 Americans were arrested in 1997 on marijuana charges, 83 percent for simple possession.

Still groups such as the Family Research Council say any easing of drug laws would send a dangerous signal, particularly to teens, that will only make a bad problem worse.

MARIJUANA LAWS SHOULD BE REFORMED

Ira Glasser

In the following selection, Ira Glasser argues that the federal government's war against marijuana violates American civil liberties. He contends that criminalizing the personal choice to use marijuana represents a gross intrusion into the private lives of American citizens. Americans who test positive for marijuana use in drug tests are losing their jobs, the author writes, and the homes and personal possessions of some Americans arrested for marijuana use are seized and sold without trial. According to Glasser, the government justifies these intrusions on the grounds that marijuana is a dangerous drug despite substantial evidence to the contrary. Glasser proposes that current laws prohibiting marijuana be reformed to protect American citizens from continued violations of their civil rights. Glasser is the executive director of the American Civil Liberties Union (ACLU), an organization dedicated to defending Americans' constitutional rights.

Before January of 1998, no one except his most devoted friends and followers had ever heard of Ross Rebagliati. But this 20-something Canadian snow boarder became an international figure after his hard-won Olympic gold medal was temporarily snatched away from him when a post-event drug screen revealed traces of marijuana metabolites in his urine. After a suspense-filled 48 hours, the Court of Arbitration of Sports decided to return the medal to its rightful owner.

The conclusion to this episode was a surprise to those who have become accustomed to defeat in the arena of marijuana law reform. Along with the passage of a medical marijuana voters' initiative in California and a more broadly worded drug reform initiative in Arizona in November 1996, it is a signal of real progress in an area that has for so long defied reform.

The marijuana issue is not new to the American Civil Liberties Union (ACLU) or its members. We have officially opposed marijuana prohibition since 1968. Since then, some things have changed, but

Excerpted from "Spotlight: Why Marijuana Law Reform Should Matter to You," by Ira Glasser, *National ACLU Members' Bulletin*, Spring 1998. Reprinted with permission from the ACLU.

too much has remained the same. In the past 30 years, 10 million people have been arrested for marijuana offenses in the U.S., the vast majority of them for possession and use. Indeed, in 1996 there were 641,600 marijuana arrests in this country, 85% of them for possession; more than in any previous year!

The hopeful news is that after being bombarded for decades with inflammatory and often false drug war rhetoric, the American public seems more receptive to marijuana law reform today than it has in many years. A strong majority has supported the legal availability of medical marijuana at least since 1995, when a poll commissioned by the ACLU revealed that 79% of the public said they thought it "would be a good idea to legalize marijuana to relieve pain and for other medical uses if prescribed by a doctor."

It's time for the ACLU to move the issue of marijuana reform front and center. During the worst excesses of the war on drugs, the silence of civil libertarians only emboldened our opponents to push through more and more draconian measures and helped create an atmosphere in which politicians were afraid to talk rationally about the marijuana issue. Recent successes have already brought about the predictable backlash, including the Clinton Administration's threat to punish California physicians who recommended marijuana to their patients. The ACLU can and should play a major role in fending off the government's efforts to undermine marijuana law reform.

Excessive Government Intrusion

Why should the ACLU and its members care about this issue? First and foremost, because it is wrong in principle for the government to criminalize such personal behavior. A government that cannot make it a crime for an individual to drink a martini should for the same reasons not be permitted to make it a crime to smoke marijuana. John Stuart Mill said it perfectly back in 1857 in his famous essay, "On Liberty": "Over himself," he wrote, "over his own body and mind, the individual is sovereign." And Americans certainly behave as if they believe that: marijuana is the third most popular drug in America after alcohol and nicotine (approximately 18 million adults used it in 1997, and 10 million are regular smokers).

The criminal prohibition of marijuana thus represents an extraordinary degree of government intrusion into the private, personal lives of those adults who choose to use it. Moreover, marijuana users are not the only victims of such a policy because a government that crosses easily over into this zone of personal behavior will cross over into others. The right to personal autonomy—what Mill called individual sovereignty—in matters of religion, political opinion, sexuality, reproductive decisions, and other private, consensual activities is at risk so long as the state thinks it can legitimately punish people for choosing a marijuana joint over a martini.

Civil Liberties Violations

Second, marijuana prohibition is the cause of a host of other very serious civil liberties violations. Millions of employees in both the public
and private sectors are now subject to urinalysis drug testing programs, whether or not they are suspected of using drugs. Marijuana is
the most common drug turned up by these "body fluid searches"
since it is used by many more people than the other illicit drugs, and
is detectable for days or weeks after ingestion (long after it has ceased
to have any psychoactive effects). A positive marijuana drug test can
lead to suspension, termination and coerced drug treatment, even
though it does not measure intoxication or impairment. It is as if you
were tested and fired from your job for a drink you had at a party last
Saturday night.

The government's seizure and civil forfeiture of people's homes,
cars and other assets on the grounds they were "used in the commission of" a marijuana offense is another egregious example. The so-
called zero tolerance policy has caused outlandishly disproportionate
penalties, like the seizure, without trial, of an automobile because a
single marijuana joint was found in the glove compartment. People's
homes and other possessions have been seized and sold, all without a
trial. Forfeiture can take place even when no criminal charges are
brought, and it is then the individual's burden to petition a court for
the return of his or her property. Often the police quickly sell the
seized asset and pocket the money for general departmental use.

Ever since 1937, when it adopted the "Marihuana Tax Act," the
government has justified the criminalization of marijuana use on the
grounds that it is a dangerous drug. But this claim looks more and
more ludicrous with each passing year. Every independent commission appointed to look into this claim has found that marijuana is relatively benign. For example, President Nixon's National Commission
on Marihuana and Drug Abuse concluded in 1972 that "there is little
proven danger of physical or psychological harm from the experimental or intermittent use of natural preparations of cannabis," and recommended that marijuana for personal use be decriminalized. Ten
years later, the National Academy of Sciences issued its finding that
"over the past forty years, marijuana has been accused of causing an
array of anti-social effects including . . . provoking crime and violence
. . . leading to heroin addiction . . . and destroying the American work
ethic in young people. [These] beliefs . . . have not been substantiated
by scientific evidence."

Now here we are in 1998 and the government, along with anti-
marijuana organizations like the Partnership for a Drug Free America,
still persist in distorting the evidence, claiming, for example, that
marijuana "kills brain cells" and that it is a "gateway" to hard drugs
like cocaine and heroin. These fear tactics are a linchpin in the gov-

ernment's effort to maintain prohibition and the civil liberties violations that flow from it.

Working for Reform

With the continued support of our members, the ACLU will play an active role in bringing about genuine marijuana law reform. Our litigation efforts to end suspicionless drug testing of workers and students, to challenge civil forfeiture laws and to defend the First Amendment right of doctors to recommend marijuana to their patients will all continue, and we hope to establish a special project in the national office to bring legal challenges against other civil liberties violations brought about by prohibition. Our lobbyists at both the state and national levels will continue to oppose repressive legislation and support reform, like Representative Barney Frank's medical marijuana bill [which would make it legal under federal law for doctors to prescribe marijuana]. And we will work hard to educate the public as well, through media relations, publications and other forms of outreach.

ACLU members, too, have a critical role to play. This is a debate that needs to take place in every community. Fundamental questions about individual freedom and limits on government power need to be addressed. You can write letters to your local newspapers and let your elected representatives at all levels know what you think.

Marijuana Should Not Be Legalized

D.S. Perez

Those who support legalization claim that marijuana is not as harmful as alcohol or other drugs, writes D.S. Perez in the following selection. However, he maintains, marijuana actually is a dangerous drug that should not be legalized for any reason, including medical use. According to Perez, if legalized, marijuana would likely be marketed by the powerful tobacco industry. As a result, he claims, marijuana use would drastically increase, compounding America's problem with addiction and contributing to the destruction of American families. Perez is a senior staff writer for the *Spartan Daily News*, a publication of San Jose State University in San Jose, California.

Sometime in the near future, the U.S. Supreme Court will bring down the judgment on the movement to make medical marijuana legal, which is the first step toward legalizing what has been an illegal drug. [The U.S. Supreme Court ruled on May 14, 2001, that California cannabis clubs may not legally distribute marijuana.]

Proponents of legalization will contend that cannabis, marijuana, hemp, weed or whatnot could stop the drug war that's not working, reduce gang violence and problems with certain third-world countries that produce the raw materials for drugs and turn a shrub plant's fiber into every possible product possible.

Yes, the war on drugs has turned into a fruitless, unsuccessful campaign.

And while it sounds like hemp, cannabis, marijuana, or whatever is better than other drugs used in the medical field, it contains some ironically harmful side effects.

In short, it would be a mistake to legalize cannabis—in any fashion.

Looking for the Truth

One has to admire the spin done by those seeking to make marijuana legal.

According to those in favor of legalization, marijuana is an inno-

Reprinted, with permission, from "Marijuana, a Poison, Should Not Be Legalized," by D.S. Perez, *Spartan Daily News*, April 30, 2001.

cent substance that is nowhere near as damaging as alcohol or other drugs, and it offers benefits to those suffering cancer.

However, spin can't hide the truth.

According to an American Cancer Society article, marijuana impairs the immune system, enhances tumor growth and causes bronchitis and lung cancer, thanks to it containing four times the amount of the carcinogenic substance known as tar, which is also used in cigarettes.

So, in order to reduce the stresses of cancer, using this drug should relieve pain while killing the patient with some other form of cancer.

So why not just legalize marijuana and drop the b.s. cover of it being the miracle drug to cure everything from glaucoma to hemorrhoids?

Again, it wouldn't be a wise idea.

A New Market for the Tobacco Industry

Marijuana, once legalized, will not be sold by Mom-and-Pop outfits out of Santa Cruz and Chico, California. Instead certain corporations will take over this new green machine.

Who are they? The same people who've been rolling smokes by the billions for years, the tobacco industry.

Who else can produce a cheap (and addictive) regular supply of smokes and turn major profits?

Who else has learned how to market products which attract those too young to use their product in order to replace the dying user population, as well as make a stinky odor-stick look cool?

Answer: Big Tobacco.

Sounds revolting, doesn't it? And face it, it would be likely for Joe Camel [a cartoon designed to sell cigarettes] to come out of retirement to promote his new product, all while the new industry says it's not being marketed toward kids.

Some will argue that marijuana can be cultivated in the home, negating those sinister fat cats, but hey, beer can be brewed at home and yet people still buy cans, cases and kegs at the store. The masses don't have the time, patience or care to give to a plant, and I've known plenty of stoners who have failed in cultivating their own crop.

On that note, the marijuana industry's public relations will be strengthened by the billions of dollars of revenue flowing in, and positive spin and "scientific studies" will continue to promote the product, as well as squelch any reports citing harmful effects in the human body or in society.

Already, a search on the *Google* search engine shows links under the American Cancer Society's article defending marijuana and denouncing these scientific claims, coming back with arguments that aren't sound.

One such Web site puts up a defense stating that everything in the world causes cancer, which may have been a defense the tobacco companies may have considered.

With marijuana legalized, use of the drug would not decrease, but rather, it would increase and the number of problems associated with it and alcohol abuse—unwanted or problematic pregnancies, suicide, homicide, domestic violence—would also rise.

You see, humans are a species of addicts. This nation alone has gambling addicts, alcoholics and people who can't stop eating, just to name a few groups. Almost each of these groups has a support group or therapy for those to cope with their addiction.

The problem? All of these groups are either too expensive or have minuscule financial backing and support. And don't think the new cannabis industry will shell out bucks for 12-step programs designed to curb its "overzealous customers."

After all, the gambling industry doesn't give much support to Gamblers Anonymous either, aside from a tiny sticker on the side of an ATM machine, and cigarette packages and alcoholic beverages have the Surgeon General's warning in small type.

Also, 12-step programs aren't always effective. Yes, there are many people who do kick their habits and hold their own, but there are many who can't discipline themselves from the urge.

It's just not right to legalize this poison. We already have alcohol and tobacco to worry about. This society needs not another poison on the market shelves where consumers can mindlessly waste their lives.

As I end this column, I have a feeling that I'm in the minority opinion.

Maybe I'm being overzealous. Maybe I'm missing the boat. Maybe I'm with the same cast-offs who crusade against abortion or eating meat.

But I just can't get what I've seen out of my mind. All of the addictions to sins in a household from hell.

I can just picture a kid living in a house where Mom's stoned so she can reduce the pain from Dad's rage when he's roaring drunk and pissed from blowing all his money on bad bets.

I can see this kid's 14-year-old sister already stealing tokes from Mom's stash of marijuana cigarettes and speed. She hasn't been to school for about a month, but nobody notices.

The power is off because no one has had the brains to pay the bill for three months, and the kitchen stinks of smoke and rotting food, and most of it is already unhealthy to eat.

And this house isn't the only one of its kind in the neighborhood.

Come to think of it, it's the house of some members of my family. And worse, I've already seen this home in real life. I stayed in those homes a few times.

I don't think anyone else has to.

RESPONSIBLE MARIJUANA USE SHOULD BE LEGAL

R. Keith Stroup

According to R. Keith Stroup, executive director of the National Organization for the Reform of Marijuana Laws (NORML), the responsible use of marijuana should be legal. In the following selection, taken from his 1997 testimony before the Committee on the Judiciary Council of the District of Columbia, Stroup explains that many middle-class Americans use marijuana as a recreational drug just as others drink alcohol or smoke cigarettes. However, Stroup argues, unlike social drinkers or tobacco smokers, people who use marijuana are treated like criminals. He maintains that singling out moderate smokers of marijuana for harsh punishment is unjust. Stroup also proposes a code of conduct for the responsible use of marijuana that would restrict its consumption to adults, prohibit marijuana-impaired driving, and discourage abuse.

Since 1970, NORML has been a voice for Americans who believe it is both counter-productive and unjust to treat marijuana smokers as criminals. Arresting and jailing otherwise law-abiding citizens who happen to be marijuana smokers serves no legitimate societal purpose. Rather it is an enormous waste of valuable law enforcement resources that should be focused on truly serious crime, and it has a terribly destructive impact on the lives, careers and families of those Americans who are arrested and jailed. We have declared war against a whole segment of our own citizens, without cause. It is time to end marijuana prohibition.

We do not suggest that marijuana is totally harmless or that it cannot be abused. That is true for all drugs, including those which are legal. We do believe that moderate marijuana use is relatively harmless—far less harmful to the user than either tobacco or alcohol, for example—and that any risk presented by marijuana smoking falls well within the ambit of choice we permit the individual in a free society. Today, far more harm is caused by marijuana prohibition than by marijuana itself.

Reprinted from R. Keith Stroup's testimony before The Committee on The Judiciary Council of the District of Columbia, May 7, 1997.

The Recreational Use of Marijuana

It's time we put to rest the myth that smoking marijuana is a fringe or deviant activity, engaged in only by those on the margins of American society. In reality, marijuana smoking is extremely common, and marijuana is the recreational drug of choice for millions of mainstream, middle class Americans. According to the most recent NIDA [National Institute on Drug Abuse] data, between 66 million Americans have smoked marijuana at some time in their lives, 18 million have smoked marijuana in the last year, and 10 million are current smokers (have smoked as at least once in the last month). In fact, NIDA found that 61% of all current illicit drug users report that marijuana is the only drug they have used; this figure rises to 80% if hashish (a marijuana derivative) is included.

A national survey of voters found that 34%—one third of the voting adults in the country—acknowledged having smoked marijuana at some point in their lives. Many successful business and professional leaders, including many state and federal elected officials from both political parties, admit they have smoked marijuana. We should begin to reflect that reality in our state and federal legislation, and stop acting as if otherwise law-abiding marijuana smokers are part of the crime problem. They are not, and it is absurd to continue to spend law enforcement resources arresting and jailing them.

Marijuana smokers in this country are no different from their non-smoking peers, except for their marijuana use. Like most Americans, they are responsible citizens who work hard, raise families, contribute to their communities, and want a safe, crime-free neighborhood in which to live. Because of our marijuana laws, these citizens face criminal arrest and imprisonment solely because they choose to smoke a marijuana cigarette when they relax, instead of drinking alcohol. They simply prefer marijuana over alcohol as their recreational drug of choice. This is a misapplication of the criminal sanction which undermines respect for the law in general and extends government into areas of our private life that are inappropriate.

The Responsible Use of Marijuana

At NORML, we believe that marijuana smokers, like those who drink alcohol, have a responsibility to behave appropriately and to assure that their recreational drug use is conducted in a responsible manner. Neither marijuana smoking nor alcohol consumption is ever an excuse for misconduct of any kind, and both smokers and drinkers must be held to the same standard as all Americans.

The NORML Board of Directors has issued the following statement entitled "Principles of Responsible Cannabis Use," which defines the conduct which we believe any responsible marijuana smoker should follow:

I. *Adults Only*

Cannabis consumption is for adults only. It is irresponsible to provide cannabis to children. Many things and activities are suitable for young people, but others absolutely are not. Children do not drive cars, enter into contracts, or marry, and they must not use drugs. As it is unrealistic to demand lifetime abstinence from cars, contracts and marriage, however, it is unrealistic to expect lifetime abstinence from all intoxicants, including alcohol. Rather, our expectation and hope for young people is that they grow up to be responsible adults. Our obligation to them is to demonstrate what that means.

II. *No Driving*

The responsible cannabis consumer does not operate a motor vehicle or other dangerous machinery impaired by cannabis, nor (like other responsible citizens) impaired by any other substance or condition, including some medicines and fatigue. Although cannabis is said by most experts to be safer than alcohol and many prescription drugs with motorists, responsible cannabis consumers never operate motor vehicles in an impaired condition. Public safety demands not only that impaired drivers be taken of the road, but that objective measures of impairment be developed and used, rather than chemical testing.

III. *Set and Setting*

The responsible cannabis user will carefully consider his/her set and setting, regulating use accordingly. "Set" refers to the consumer's values, attitudes, experience and personality, and "setting" means the consumer's physical and social circumstances. The responsible cannabis consumer will be vigilant as to conditions—time, place, mood, etc.—and does not hesitate to say "no" when those conditions are not conducive to a safe, pleasant and/or productive experience.

IV. *Resist Abuse*

Use of cannabis, to the extent that it impairs health, personal development or achievement, is abuse, to be resisted by responsible cannabis users. Abuse means harm. Some cannabis use is harmful; most is not. That which is harmful should be discouraged; that which is not need not be. Wars have been waged in the name of eradicating "drug abuse", but instead of focusing on abuse, enforcement measures have been diluted by targeting all drug use, whether abusive or not. If marijuana abuse is to be targeted, it is essential that clear standards be developed to identify it.

V. *Respect Rights of Others*

The responsible cannabis user does not violate the rights of others, observes accepted standards of courtesy and public propriety, and respects the preferences of those who wish to avoid cannabis entirely. No one may violate the rights of others, and no substance use excuses any such violation. Regardless of the legal status of cannabis, responsible users will adhere to emerging tobacco smoking protocols in public and private places. As these principles indicate, we believe there is a difference between use and abuse, and the government should limit its involvement and concentrate its resources to discourage irresponsible marijuana use. Responsible marijuana use causes no harm to society and should be of no interest to the government in a free society.

Stop Arresting Marijuana Smokers

The "war on drugs" is not really about drugs; if it were, tobacco and alcohol would be your primary targets. They are the most commonly used and abused drugs in America and unquestionably they cause far more harm to the user and to society than does marijuana. Instead, the war on drugs has become a war on marijuana smokers, and in any war there are casualties. According to the latest FBI statistics, in 1995 nearly one-half million (489,000) Americans were arrested on marijuana charges. That is the largest number of marijuana arrests ever made in this country in any single year, and reflects a 70% increase over 1991 (288,000). Eighty-six percent (86%) of those arrests were for possession, not sale.

Those were real people who were paying taxes, supporting their families, and working hard to make a better life for their children; suddenly they are arrested and jailed and treated as criminals, solely because they smoke marijuana. This is a travesty of justice that causes enormous pain, suffering and financial hardship for millions of American families. It also engenders disrespect for the law and for the criminal justice system overall. Responsible marijuana smokers present no threat or danger to America, and there is no reason to treat them as criminals. As a society we need to find ways to discourage personal conduct of all kinds that is abusive or harmful to others. Responsible marijuana smokers are not the problem and it's time to stop arresting them.

It's time to seek a policy that minimizes the harm associated with marijuana smoking and marijuana prohibition—a policy that distinguishes between use and abuse, and reflects the importance we have always attached in this country to the right of the individual to be free from the overreaching power of government. Most of us would agree the government has no business knowing what books we read, the subject of our telephone conversations, or how we conduct ourselves in the privacy of our bedroom. Similarly, whether we smoke marijuana or drink alcohol to relax is simply not an appropriate area of concern for the government.

By stubbornly defining all marijuana smoking as criminal, including that which involves adults smoking in the privacy of their home, we are wasting police and prosecutorial resources, clogging courts, filling costly and scarce jail and prison space, and needlessly wrecking the lives and careers of genuinely good citizens. It's time we ended marijuana prohibition and stopped arresting and jailing hundreds of thousands of average Americans whose only "crime" is that they smoke marijuana. This is a tragic and senseless war against our own citizens; it must be ended.

LEGALIZING MARIJUANA WOULD BE IRRESPONSIBLE

Lee P. Brown

The following selection is taken from a keynote address delivered by Lee P. Brown at the National Conference on Marijuana Use in 1995. According to Brown, advocates of the legalization of marijuana are evading their responsibility to protect America's young people. Marijuana is not the harmless substance those who support legalization would lead Americans to believe, Brown argues, yet popular culture continues to glamorize marijuana use and imply that smoking marijuana is "cool." Brown claims that Americans have a moral duty to let young people know that marijuana is dangerous and to promote a drug-free society. At the time that this speech was given, Brown was the director of the Office of National Drug Control Policy.

Let me begin by thanking Dr. Alan Leshner, Director of the National Institute on Drug Abuse, and Donna Shalala, Secretary of Health and Human Services, for inviting me to participate in this most important conference.

I want to commend Dr. Leshner and Secretary Shalala for their leadership in making this conference a reality. As the first national conference to focus on providing scientifically based information on marijuana, this effort is significant because we will have the opportunity to shatter some long-lingering myths about marijuana while at the same time providing a wakeup call to the Nation.

This wakeup call is all important. We who have access to the most accurate and advanced information should be driving the discussion about finding solutions to the drug problem, not those with the least knowledge who often seem to have the most to say.

Sending the Wrong Message

For instance, outside of this hotel today are protesters and demonstrators who advocate the legalization of drugs in this society. At a time when every indicator points to an upsurge in drug use among our youngsters, how responsible is it for any adult to advance the message that using drugs is okay?

Reprinted from Lee P. Brown's Keynote Address to the National Conference on Marijuana Use: Prevention, Treatment and Research, July 19, 1995.

Even the Speaker of the House—Newt Gingrich—has gotten into the act. He [has] said that the choice about the Nation's drug problem is to "Either legalize it or get rid of it." Mr. Gingrich's statement is the ultimate in extremism and defeatism. Drug abuse is an American crisis, not a partisan political opportunity. It does not help kids or serve them well when our leaders play partisan politics with an issue that goes to the heart of everything we hold dear.

If we care about our children, we must treat drug use as the threat that it is. President [Bill] Clinton and I are committed to fighting this threat with all the resources available to us. You will not hear us playing politics with the lives of American youngsters. And you will never hear us talking about legalization. Anyone who advocates that we legalize drugs has abdicated responsibility. Today, I urge the Speaker of the House and his colleagues to work together with us to implement the President's antidrug strategy instead of pretending they have a simplistic silver bullet that they know will not work.

Substance abuse is a serious matter. It claims the lives of many Americans each year. It touches all of us in one way or another. If a family member is an abuser, the whole family suffers. When families suffer, so, too, does the community. And when communities are in need, the whole Nation must stop and take notice. Substance abuse costs this Nation millions of dollars in lost revenues each year. The costs associated with incarceration, criminal case processing, victimization, accidents, and lost property due to substance abuse and related crime total more than $67 million annually.

Creating a Drug-Free Society

So, it is clear that when we come together to discuss substance abuse, whether we are talking cocaine, heroin, inhalants, or marijuana, we are talking about one of the most critical issues of our time. President Clinton and I are committed to making America a drug-free society. We are committed to saving our young people from the dangers of drug use and drug trafficking. We will do whatever it takes to make this a reality across this land, but we cannot do this job alone.

Each of us must commit to helping our youngsters resist the lure of drugs. Each of us must demand that our schools be drug-free and violence-free so that they can once again become the havens for learning that schools were intended to be. Each of us must make it clear that the only worthwhile drug message is a "no use" message. We cannot give mixed messages and come down hard on some drugs and soft-pedal the dangers of others.

Marijuana is a dangerous and harmful drug. We know this is true, so let's say it every chance that we get. Our young people watch us and listen to us. When we tell them that we will not tolerate any drug use, we have to make it clear that marijuana is included in this prohibition.

I have read that some baby boomer parents are ambivalent about the "no use" message when it comes to marijuana, because they do not want to appear hypocritical. Let me warn you that hypocrisy is not the issue. Keeping our youngsters safe and free from harm is. This means that we cannot equivocate on this all-important message. It has to be clear and precise—all drugs are harmful; all drugs are dangerous.

The Dangers of Using Marijuana

Marijuana is the most widely used illicit drug in America today, and this has been the case for some years. Nearly 70 million Americans have used marijuana in their lifetime. Marijuana is a potent, intoxicating drug with long-term, cumulative effects. Unlike alcohol or most other substances of abuse, it remains in the body for many hours, sometimes for a period of days. Heavy users can test positive for the drug even after weeks of abstinence.

We also need to realize that much of the marijuana that is being consumed today is far more potent than it ever was in the 1960s and 1970s, when popular culture considered it a relatively benign substance. The result is higher levels of intoxication by users, over longer periods of time, with far greater consequences.

A key indicator is the number of persons seeking hospital emergency room treatment for marijuana effects. And this number has increased dramatically in recent years. In fact, in a trend that started in 1990, marijuana-related emergencies jumped by 86 percent in the 3 years for which we now have data (through 1993).

A closer look at these figures is even more revealing. In the 12-to-17 age group, what could be described as our newest users, there were twice as many marijuana-related emergency room cases in 1993 as in 1990, when this upsurge began. Half of all marijuana emergency room cases happen to individuals under age 26.

In fact, in that same 12-to-17 age group, the youngest and newest users, marijuana now accounts for more than twice the number of hospital emergency room cases as cocaine and heroin combined. In 1993, there were 4,293 marijuana mentions in the 12-to-17 age group, 1,583 cocaine mentions, and 282 heroin-related cases. Also significant is the trend of change beginning in 1990: while marijuana use has doubled, cocaine cases among our young have gone down. Maybe the message has been heard about the dangers of cocaine.

Now it is time that this same message be heard loud and clear about marijuana. And the message is that marijuana is not benign, it is not harmless, it should not be legalized. It is a very dangerous drug that can well cause you to fight for your health and your very life in a hospital emergency room.

Another issue is the strong link between marijuana use and violence. The Parent Resource Institute for Drug Education, known as PRIDE, has studied the correlation between violent behavior and drug use and found that 66 percent of high school students who carried guns to school also used marijuana. Another important message to our youngsters is that if you use marijuana, you could end up in a violent fight, in a traffic accident, and, as we said earlier, in the hospital emergency room.

Protecting Young People

Contrary to popular opinion, marijuana does have addictive properties. The consequences of heavy use include both physical and psychological dependence. Youngsters are being misled and misinformed about the dangers of marijuana. I held a press conference on Monday, [July 17, 1995,] where we highlighted what I call the seductive marketing of American youngsters. You would be shocked at the kinds of products that are being marketed to children that glamorize drug use and getting high.

These products, which include T-shirts, bottles, gum, cigar blunts, and posters, are an initiation to a culture that implicitly sends a message that being cool is everything and that playing it safe is for losers. We have to stop Corporate America from marketing "coolness." We have to stop those who would profit at our children's expense. Kids who do not want to use drugs must not be made the targets of unscrupulous marketers.

The good news is that many of our young people already know that using marijuana is the wrong choice. Some have even spoken out saying that something has to be done about the drug use of their friends. A recent poll of student leaders revealed that many youngsters are happy that some limits are being set.

One student said, "I talked to a kid about 2 weeks ago, and he could not hold a sentence together because of drug use. I mean that was like living proof. It's like he's still on the trip he did not come back from."

Some of these same students applauded the Supreme Court's recent ruling on drug testing for high school athletes. In fact, *USA Today* reported that many of the students surveyed felt that the ruling should apply to all students, not just athletes. One female student said, "I wish something would happen in my town. Half of our soccer team smoke marijuana and drink every weekend. They need to be tested."

It is important that we recognize that not all of our youngsters are enamored with drug use. In fact, the Monitoring the Future Study reports that 61 percent of high school seniors say they have never used marijuana. What we need to do is target those youngsters who have not gotten the message. They need our help. And they need it now. . . .

Controlling Marijuana Use

Seizure, eradication, and law enforcement activity represent a significant effort to disrupt the flow of marijuana to our neighborhoods and communities. We know we have to make it more difficult for drug trafficking organizations to acquire, transport, and sell their product. These efforts, ultimately, impact the price of marijuana on the street and reduce its availability to those wishing to purchase it.

But let me emphasize that law enforcement and eradication are just two pieces of the puzzle. We also need to fund treatment for those addicted to drugs and to keep hardcore drug users off the street. We also desperately need to fund prevention programs that target potential drug users before they even begin.

Only through a concerted effort combining law enforcement, treatment, and prevention can we ever hope to really make an impact on the rate of current drug use in America. We need programs that are community-based if we are to have a fighting chance to defeat drugs, because we cannot win the fight against drugs and crime with Federal initiatives alone. This is a long-term problem that will yield only to long-term commitment. I urge all of you to come together in your communities to change the social environment for all who live there.

And finally, I need you, as the experts in the field, to help me in our crusade against dangerous drugs. The country needs you to spread the word to parents and children about the work that you are doing. Your presence here today means you understand the importance of outreach. Let everyone—parents, children, the media, everyone you know—understand what your research and your community efforts have found about the dangers of marijuana.

Use your knowledge and position to urge parents in your communities to talk to their children about marijuana and about all drug use. Tell your friends to stay informed and clear about what is acceptable behavior and what is not.

Let your own children know that because they matter so much, you care so much about their well-being and safety. Ask them to carry this message, to become leaders in school in the antidrug effort.

In short, we all have to let children know that we care. And because we care, we need them to know that drugs are wrong and they are dangerous. This is a message about the future of our country. If we fail at this, we fail our children and our communities, and the whole society will suffer.

But I am very hopeful about our future generation. There are enough youngsters in America who want to do the right thing. We have to guide them and provide a safe passage. It is a moral duty, my friends, that I am talking about.

Join me in this crusade to make our country drug-free so that our children can grow and develop healthy in body and spirit.

The Movement to Legalize Industrial Hemp

Mari Kane

In the following selection, Mari Kane explains that industrial hemp was virtually prohibited by the Marijuana Tax Act of 1937, which did not distinguish between hemp and marijuana. The two come from the same plant, Kane writes, but hemp does not have the psychoactive ingredient found in marijuana and therefore cannot be used to produce a high. Instead, she reports, industrial hemp is a versatile fiber that has the potential to become a very valuable agricultural crop. Kane admits that some people fear the movement to legalize industrial hemp is actually headed by pro-marijuana activists who promote recreational drug use. However, she contends that many mainstream farmers and entrepreneurs are leading advocates of the hemp industry. Kane is a hemp advocate and publisher of *The Industrial Hemp Journal* and *Hemp Pages: The Hemp Industry Source Book*.

After 60 years as a pariah plant, sprayed into oblivion by federal agents wherever it appeared, the versatile fiber known as industrial hemp appears to be making a dramatic comeback, with legalization movements in 14 states, and, in North Dakota, an outright victory. Will hemp, the fiber that helped win World War II, finally emerge from the dark shadow of its close relative, marijuana?

The History of Hemp

Growing hemp was by no means always illegal in the United States. In the 18th century, hemp was such a valued commodity, in shipping and other industries, that Thomas Jefferson, then ambassador to France, smuggled illegally obtained Chinese hemp seeds to the colonies. Those same seeds were eventually hybridized to create the famous Kentucky Hemp strain. George Washington even said, in a letter to his farm manager, "make the most you can of the Indian hemp seed. Sow it everywhere."

It's true that hemp and marijuana come from the same plant—Cannabis sativa L. It's not true that the plants are the same. The biological difference between them is demonstrated by their respective levels of tetrahydrocannabinol (THC), the plant's psychoactive ingredient. For industrial hemp, the generally accepted THC level is one percent or less; for recreational marijuana, the THC level is at least three percent. The physical differences between the two plants are readily apparent. Hemp grows lean and tall with flowers on the canopy; marijuana branches widely with resinous buds on all sides.

Until the early 1900s, cannabis hemp was treated like any other farm crop and its cultivation required no special regulations or licenses. Hundreds of thousands of acres of hemp grew in Kentucky, Tennessee, Iowa, Nebraska, South Dakota, Wisconsin, Minnesota and Michigan.

Then, in 1931, the nation's first drug czar, Harry Anslinger, was appointed to head the newly reorganized Federal Bureau of Narcotic and Dangerous Drugs by his future uncle-in-law and the Secretary of the Treasury, Andrew Mellon. At the time, the Mellon Bank of Pittsburgh was the chief financial backer for DuPont, the munitions and plastics maker, a company which viewed recent technological advances in hemp processing as a threat.

Anslinger took his job very seriously and molded himself after J. Edgar Hoover of the FBI. He hired ex-G-men, newly unemployed after Prohibition ended in 1929, and created an army of officers to fight the nation's first Drug War. In only a few years, public vice number one went from being alcohol to cannabis. The drug's role as "Assassin of Youth" was reflected in period films like the camp classic *Reefer Madness*.

In 1937, *Popular Mechanics* declared hemp to be the "New Billion Dollar Crop" because of new developments in fiber technology. Also in 1937, the ever-fervent Harry Anslinger introduced the Marijuana Prohibitive Tax Act, proposing an excise tax on dealers and a transfer tax on sales. After hearing Anslinger testify under oath that "marijuana is the most violence-causing drug in the history of mankind," and against the protests of the American Medical Association, the National Oilseed Institute and the birdseed industry, the Marijuana Tax Act was passed by Congress. Anslinger assured the legislators that farmers "could go on growing hemp much as they always have."

Hemp farmers lined up for licenses and received $1 Special Tax Stamps. Now hemp was regulated by the Treasury Department and, in some states, the farmers were harassed by federal agents. Eventually, and in spite of the brief World War II "Hemp for Victory" campaign, hemp fell out of vogue in the domestic market, and 1957 saw the last American hemp harvest. Stands of wild hemp that still grow across the plains states serve as gentle reminders of America's once-vital hemp culture.

Although hemp cultivation is not technically illegal, farmers need a license to grow it. But if the agency in charge of licensing refuses to issue a permit, you could be prosecuted for growing hemp. When the federal government began issuing Marijuana Tax Stamps in 1938, jurisdiction over both hemp and marijuana fell into the hands of the Federal Bureau of Narcotics, now the Drug Enforcement Agency (DEA), which lumped both into Schedule One of the federal list of controlled substances. By the agency's rules, hemp has "a high potential for abuse."

An Arduous Climb

Despite its outlaw status, hemp is slowly climbing back into favor as a base for a huge variety of consumer products, from clothing to ice cream. Thousands of hemp businesses have risen (and sometimes fallen) since 1993. Estimates of national and international sales of hemp goods in 1997 range from $50 million to $100 million. After a decade of public re-education, most people know the difference between industrial hemp and marijuana.

Currently, 99.9 percent of industrial hemp used in the United States is imported from Eastern Europe, China and Canada. Goods made from imported raw materials are expensive, and most experts acknowledge that for the American hemp industry to succeed financially, there must be a domestic, bioregional source of hemp seed and fiber. Sixty years after the Marijuana Tax Act, though, the domestic hemp industry's growth is still stymied by drug war politics. Bill Clinton, the self-acknowledged pot-smoking president, has actually increased the federal drug budget to an unprecedented $18 billion per year, primarily to fight marijuana production.

In 1996, the anti-drug community woke up to the growing interest in industrial hemp. That year, then-drug czar Lee Brown attempted to publicly shame shoemaking giant Adidas out of naming its tennis shoe "The Hemp." But 1996 was also the year Californians voted in favor of Prop 215, virtually decriminalizing use of marijuana for medical purposes. The feds, worried about the growing legitimization of all forms of the hemp plant, threatened to pull the DEA licenses of doctors who recommended cannabis to patients, thus disabling them from prescribing medications. The White House Office of National Drug Policy announced that "hemp sends the wrong messages to children." Other standard lines: "law enforcement officers can't tell the difference between hemp and marijuana" or, despite obvious physical differences between the two plants, "marijuana could be hidden in a hemp field."

The hemp industry's response to hemp field marijuana is that it's not practical, because the process by which industrial hemp plants shed pollen means that any nearby marijuana plant would lose quality. Theoretically, fields of industrial hemp could be the best marijuana eradication device ever conceived. Still, money earmarked for cannabis suppression is being used to destroy wild hemp. The Vermont legislature's 1998 study of the $500 million DEA Cannabis Eradication and

Suppression Program showed that 99.28 percent of the 422,716,526 hemp plants confiscated were actually wild hemp, descendants of a bygone industrial era.

Strange Bedfellows

The altruistic, right-livelihood "Hemp Movement" is ailing. Replacing the hippie hempsters is a corporate culture that includes venture capital and public trading. Nobody works for "the cause" anymore. One might suppose that with an adversary as large and parochial as Uncle Sam, the hemp industry would work to be as united as possible, but that's not the case. Industrial hemp offers the lure of financial gain, and this has turned some would-be entrepreneurs against each other.

North America's hemp industry today is composed of basically two sets of interests: the hempsters, the visionaries who turned a cottage industry into a major business, and who have maintained a 300-member trade organization called the Hemp Industries Association (HIA); and the "hemp suits," a loose affiliation of bureaucrats, entrepreneurs, academics and farmers who plan to take the industry into the future. They have formed a 60-member association called the North American Industrial Hemp Alliance (NAIHC).

Conflicts between the hemp groups have sometimes led to political stalemates. One glaring example is the situation in California, the first state to decriminalize medical use of marijuana, and the place where the hemp industry was born. A fledgling organization, Californians for Industrial Renewal (CAIR) is the only group working to legalize hemp on the state level. CAIR got its start with an unsuccessful referendum to decriminalize hemp in 1998. NAIHC stayed away. NAIHC Secretary John Roulac says CAIR miscalculated by allowing only a few months to gather the required voter signatures. "It was too little, too late," he says.

One year later, the big money is still not betting on legalization, despite the fact that, in March 1999, the state assembly adopted a pro-hemp resolution. CAIR founder Sam Clauter of Orange County has been able to raise only a few thousand dollars toward a legislative campaign, and has had a variety of doors slammed in his face. "The hemp people can only donate some of their products, the farmers think I'm into drug policy reform and the foundation people think I don't push drug policy reform enough!" Clauter says with some exasperation. He is spending his own money on the campaign, which averages $1,000 a month in expenses.

One would think that Hollywood money would flow for this cause. But hemp's favorite son, California resident Woody Harrelson, has for the past four years invested his money not in California, but in Kentucky, the home state of his friend, Joe Hickey.

Hickey is the executive director of the Kentucky Hemp Growers Collective, a co-op consisting of tobacco farmers whose fathers and grandfathers once grew hemp. Harrelson very publicly planted four hemp seeds in a Kentucky field to challenge what he called an overly broad state ban covering all parts of the hemp plant. Harrelson's case has been won, appealed, and now is being considered by Kentucky's Supreme Court. The legal costs have run into the hundreds of thousands of dollars. "It's too bad I can't get funding, because the most potential for progress is here in California," laments Clauter. "It has the biggest agricultural base, the most political clout and economic influence."

An Uneasy Alliance

The hemp camps coexist in a fragile and uneasy alliance. Six years into the movement, "Rope vs. Dope" remains the dominant debate. While most in the hemp industry agree that the issues of industrial hemp and the controversial medical use of marijuana should be kept strictly separate, there is much dissent over how far this separation should go, considering the politics involved. "I think the two issues should be separate, but let's not be hypocritical," says Carolyn Moran, founder of Living Tree Paper Company and HIA board member. "This kind of division is unfair to sick people. We need to support medical use, whether we are on the right, left, or in between."

Hempsters have always been pegged by policy makers as legalizers in hemp clothing. Some hempsters did come from backgrounds in marijuana activism, others from self-employment. Hemp suits must constantly be on their guard about fraternizing with hempsters. Any relationship can come back to haunt them, as it did in 1997 when a suit-wearing hemp lobbyist in Missouri was exposed as on the payroll of the magazine *High Times*, which advocates legalizing marijuana. As a result, former general Barry McCaffrey, head of the Clinton administration's Office of National Drug Policy, wrote to all local farm bureau presidents, encouraging them to oppose hemp. That prompted the Missouri Farm Bureau to drop its hemp endorsement and, one month later, the American Farm Bureau followed suit. It was an embarrassing setback.

The NAIHC was created as a counterculture-free zone for tobacco farmers and other mainstream hemp advocates. The chairman of the NAIHC board, "Bud" Sholts, is a former official at the Wisconsin Department of Agriculture, and he recently brought ex-CIA Director James Woolsey on board as a consultant. Sholts says that Woolsey "supports the NAIHC for educational and information purposes and went with us in April to meet with McCaffrey." At that meeting, Sholts says that McCaffrey finally "got it" about the differences between hemp and marijuana. But, as a 501(c)(3) organization, Sholts insists, "the NAIHC doesn't do lobbying."

After three years of research cultivation, Canada is now in its second year of commercial growing. Its main market is the United States, where a plethora of manufacturers eagerly await arrivals of fresh seed and fiber from contractors north of the border. Unlike the European Union, Canada offers no subsidies to hemp farmers, but does require a labyrinthian application process described by 1998's farmers as "a nightmare." American hemp farmers are similarly not expecting to receive subsidies for a crop they've had to fight so hard to grow.

Reaching a consensus on industrial hemp's profitability is difficult, but some figures do exist. In 1997, Kentucky hemp farmers commissioned a study of the hemp market by the Department of Business and Economics at the University of Kentucky. It concluded that a crop of hemp seed, or grain, and straw could bring a return of as much as $319.51 per acre, compared with $135.84 per acre for white corn.

Inevitably though, the price of raw hemp will plummet once processing technology gets up to speed and when the supply meets demand. The question of the day is: how far can farm prices drop while still being profitable and attractive to farmers? Already, the cost of imported hemp is two to three times more than the substances it replaces. Although, as a premium fiber, hemp should not be compared with cotton and wood pulp, manufacturers will still need a 20 to 40 percent reduction to be able to sell mass quantities of food, body care products, paper and clothes at affordable price points.

Despite these variables, many tobacco farmers are clamoring to grow hemp. The reason, says Kentucky farmer Andy Graves, is that "tobacco is a shrinking market, and it's a dying industry. Every time the price of a pack of cigarettes goes up, more people quit."

Along with the Community Farm Alliance in Kentucky, Dorothy Robertson is investigating hemp as a supplement or alternative to tobacco crops across the South. "One of the beautiful things about hemp is that you don't need pesticides or herbicides," Robertson says. "The plant grows so close together that it shades out all of the weeds. It's a great rotation crop because after one year you could come back with another crop and you wouldn't have the weed problem."

Hemp may actually raise the yields of succeeding crops, such as corn or soybeans, thanks to its rich leaf mold, which is 50 percent nitrogen, and its long fibrous tap roots, which aerate the soil, improve water balance and add nutrients. In the Netherlands, winter wheat yields went up 10 percent after a hemp rotation. And hemp can be grown naturally almost anywhere—including all 50 states. Less fertilizer, less agricultural chemicals, higher yields and a burgeoning market, all add up to potentially higher net incomes for farmers.

Unfortunately, hemp production would be a boon to corporate seed producers as well, such as Monsanto and Cargill, since hemp regulation will require the use of certified low-THC hemp seeds. These soon-to-be patented seeds are expected to be bio-engineered with THC chemicals removed, and "terminator" components added so that farmers cannot reproduce it year after year.

Requirements for extremely low THC levels in hemp may also lead to the monopolization of the seed market by federally-sanctioned producers, as is the case in France. Another uncertainty is whether farmers will suffer confiscation of the resulting crop or prosecution if the plant shows THC levels higher than the 0.3 percent that is likely to be adopted. Welcome to the brave new world of hemp growing.

Passing State Legislation

Getting hemp laws changed has been long and slow coming. First, there was the Colorado Hemp Initiative of 1995, sponsored by Colorado Senator Lloyd Casey. That bill, as well as the 1996 and 1997 bills, failed due to law enforcement opposition. The Colorado efforts called for commercial production of hemp and defined low-THC cannabis as it was originally intended in the 1937 Tax Act. This laid the foundation for all the other hemp legislation.

Senator Casey retired from office in 1998 and was disappointed when fellow Senator Kay Alexander refused to sponsor the bill in his absence. "Kay told me the reason she backed off was that several sheriffs in her district threatened to pull support of her," says Casey. Although Colorado did not push hemp legislation in 1998, a handful of other states did, and some laws were passed. However, those bills called for feasibility studies rather than field tests or commercial production.

In 1999, hemp legislation was introduced in 14 states: Hawaii, Illinois, Iowa, Maryland, Minnesota, Montana, New Hampshire, New Mexico, North Dakota, Oregon, Tennessee, Vermont, Virginia and Wisconsin. So far, seven states have successfully passed some kind of hemp legislation: North Dakota, Hawaii, Illinois, Virginia, New Mexico, and Minnesota. However, only the laws in North Dakota, Minnesota and Hawaii call for hemp to actually be put in the ground.

In a stunning landslide, North Dakota passed its bill, which was motivated primarily by farmers, not activists. The wording of House Bill 1428, sponsored by Rep. Monson, simply states: "Any person in this state may plant, grow, harvest, possess, process, sell, and buy industrial hemp." How did North Dakota pull it off? "Maybe it's just some karma coming together," jokes Clare Carlson, the Agricultural Policies Director and Legislative Liaison at the governor's office. "Manitoba, to the North, is ahead of us with hemp and there might be some cross-pollination going on." Carlson says that no hemp will be planted in 1999, because federal law still supersedes state law. "It's up to others to change federal policy, and we advocate using state law to leverage the feds," he says.

Hawaii's House Bill 32 authorizes privately funded industrial hemp seed variety trials in Hawaii once the state and DEA permits are issued. This program will include any entity with the cash to spend. In a letter to Hawaii Representative Cynthia Thielen, DEA Chief of Operations Gregory Williams said that ". . . DEA will consider setting the level of THC content for Cannabis sativa L., hemp that may be grown for industrial purposes." Thielen enthuses, "This is bureau-cratese for saying they are working on changing their regulations so industrial hemp can be grown again in the U.S.A."

One would expect that anything to do with hemp in Minnesota would be quickly signed into law by Jesse "the pro-hemp governor" Ventura. Minnesota House File 1238, which authorized the commis-sioner of agriculture to permit experimental plots of industrial hemp, was, however, killed in committee. But as part of an appropriations bill signed by Ventura on May 25, 1999, the state will submit an application for federal permits needed to authorize the growing of experimental hemp plots. "It was an uphill battle, but in the end I was able to persuade my colleagues to include this provision in the bill," says Representative Phyllis Kahn. "The bill that Governor Ven-tura signed into law is the first step toward the legalization of hemp."

Other bills either demand a federal change or call for paper studies:

- Illinois Senate Resolution 49 and House Resolution 168 create the Industrial Hemp Investigative and Advisory Task Force, consisting of the Director of Agriculture or a designee and 12 committee members.
- New Mexico's House Bill 104, sponsored by Representative Pauline K. Gubbel, calls for an appropriation of $50,000 for New Mexico State University to study industrial hemp as a commercial crop.
- Montana's House Resolution 2 is somewhat more assertive by requesting that the federal government officially define "hemp" as having less than one percent THC. The bill also calls for hemp to be regulated by the Department of Agriculture.
- Similarly, Virginia's House Joint Resolution 94 "memorializes" the Secretary of Agriculture, the Director of the Drug Enforce-ment Administration, and the Director of the Office of National Drug Control Policy to permit the controlled, experimental culti-vation of industrial hemp in Virginia.

High Times for Hemp

On the federal side, a March 1998 petition filed by Ralph Nader's Resource Conservation Alliance (RCA) and the NAIHC attempts to force the DEA to remove hemp from its list of federally controlled sub-stances. The agency is required to respond within a reasonable amount of time, but had not done so after 18 months [on December 19, 2000, the DEA denied the petition]. If DEA does not comply, the matter is bound for the courts. RCA's Ned Day believes that the DEA is dragging its feet out of fear. "I think they are very worried about what the states are doing," he says. "They don't want middle America coming after them, especially soccer moms. It might be that they'll wait until the pressure dies down and if they feel they have cover, they might act."

Native Americans should technically be able to grow hemp since their reservations are sovereign nations—a theory which is now being tested. Since 1997, the Lakota Sioux at Pine Ridge Reservation in South Dakota have been passing ordinances and resolutions to grow hemp. In 1999, the tribe planted approximately two acres next to a field of wild hemp growing along a creek. So far, there's been no reaction from the DEA.

The Lakota are also planning construction of homes made from hemp bricks. The tribe is hoping to use part of the $5 million in federal funds it's receiving to replace 25 homes recently destroyed by tornadoes for hemp buildings. "The whole housing scene is in flux here," says tribal spokesman Tom Cook. "With all these houses going down, hemp is the only thing going up."

Meanwhile, the American Farm Bureau now has no official policy on hemp. Dave Kelly, the bureau's assistant director of news services, says, "Hemp is an issue our delegates have determined they want to be neutral on; not for it, not against it."

Signs of Light

Will the legalizing states get away with growing a crop that the federal government still considers a Schedule One restricted substance? In the DEA's letter to Hawaii's Thielen, Williams noted "that public and commercial interest may be better served if the cultivation of Cannabis sativa L. hemp is authorized by the appropriate Federal and State entities."

In line with the DEA, the White House drug czar, General McCaffrey, appears to be softening his stance. "If people believe that hemp fiber can be sold in the marketplace for a profit, and aren't actually trying to normalize the growing of marijuana around America, to the extent you want to grow hemp fiber we'd be glad to work with you," he said in April 1999. "[But as a profitable crop] I think it's going nowhere." A growing hemp industry, poised for legalization, might disagree.

THE HEMP MOVEMENT: A DISGUISE FOR LEGALIZING MARIJUANA

Jeanette McDougal

Many of those who support the hemp movement also advocate the legalization of marijuana and other drugs, writes Jeanette McDougal in the following selection. For example, she cites the editors of the pro-marijuana magazine *High Times*, who maintain that the legalization of hemp products will lead to the eventual acceptance of recreational marijuana use. McDougal also lists several members of the North American Industrial Hemp Council, pointing out their ties to organizations that work for legalization of marijuana. Furthermore, the author notes that hemp is not the profitable crop that many farmers had hoped it would be. McDougal is a teacher in St. Paul, Minnesota, and chair of Drug Watch International's hemp committee.

Separating hemp reality from hemp rhetoric is like separating fleas from dogs: It's hard to do, and it's temporary. When one hemp fact is established, pro-hemp advocates rush in with another of their own facts. Should we really turn for facts to former CIA Director James Woolsey, who bragged about his client the North American Industrial Hemp Council, by saying there was not a tie-dyed shirt owner among the members? He neglected to check their boxers. Several of the board members were either vigorous pro-drug advocates or their close associates.

A Cover for Legalizing Pot

David Morris, former vice-president of the council, pushed legalization of marijuana, marijuana cigarettes for medicine and industrial cannabis hemp for years in his columns in the St. Paul (Minn.) *Pioneer Press*.

Andrew Graves, founding and former board member, was party to a lawsuit to permit the growing of industrial cannabis hemp. The two lead lawyers in that suit—Michael Kennedy of New York and Burl McCoy of Kentucky—are on the roster of the National Organization for Reform of Marijuana Laws, an aggressive pro-marijuana legalization advocate.

Actor Woody Harrelson, an admitted pot smoker, marijuana and hemp advocate, hired Joe Hickey, executive director of the Kentucky Hemp Growers Association, as a consultant, allowing Hickey to leave his former job and devote all his time to hemp. Harrelson has sponsored many Kentucky hemp events, including a hemp essay contest for Kentucky schoolchildren, some of whom received a list of hemp facts intermingled with marijuana facts, such as, "smoking marijuana can be beneficial for emphysema, and can be used as a handy way to induce dry mouth before dental operations."

John Howell, former hemp editor of *High Times* magazine, was in Kentucky in 1998 to help Graves, Kennedy and McCoy publicize the message that there is a hemp market. Howell recently represented the cannabis hemp industry at the National Conference of State Legislatures, without disclosing his ties to *High Times*.

High Times, one of the oldest and most militant pro-drug/marijuana publications in the United States, announced in its March 1990 edition an "extraordinary plan" to legalize marijuana:

"The way to legalize marijuana is to sell marijuana legally. When you can buy marijuana in your neighborhood shopping mall, it's legal. . . . Anything and everything you can think of will be made from hemp. . . . Supporters of the hemp legalization movement will be able to buy shares in hemp manufacturing. . . . Legal and financial recognition of hemp's industrial value will mean legal marijuana, whether our government likes it or not! Pot will be legal! . . . So invest in our future. Buy some legal marijuana. Buy a hemp shirt and wear it proudly!"

Hemp's Economic Risks

As to the economics of cannabis hemp, in 1999 about 540 Canadian farmers planted 35,000 acres of hemp. About 18,700 of those acres were contracted to a company called Consolidated Growers, which went bankrupt (Chapter 7) in February 2000, leaving 232 Canadian farmers (almost half of those who planted hemp that year) holding the hemp bag for $5 million to $6 million. Much of the 1999 crop is still being stored by Canadian farmers.

In 2000, in all of Canada, a mere 13,500 acres were planted, down from 35,000 the year before. Ontario, the only province to do a costs/return per acre analysis, discovered that for fiber only, there was a $107 loss; for grain only, a $24 loss; and for grain and fiber, a $48 profit. An agriculture ministry official also warned farmers to have a contract with a reputable company before planting hemp, or they could lose $600 an acre.

The U.S. Department of Agriculture says the market for hemp fibers "will likely remain a small, thin market." The report calculates that U.S. imports of hemp fiber, yarn, fabric and seed in 1999 could have been produced on less than 5,000 acres.

The hemp liability list goes on and on and on.

THE EUROPEAN ATTITUDE TOWARD MARIJUANA

Peter Ford

Many European countries take a different approach toward marijuana than does the United States, writes Peter Ford in the following selection. He explains that several European governments have decriminalized the personal use of small amounts of marijuana or have liberalized laws dealing with marijuana offenders. For example, the Dutch government permits coffee shops to sell marijuana, Ford states, while other European countries rarely prosecute cases in which small quantities of cannabis are involved. However, he reports, most European nations continue to discourage young people from using marijuana and support programs to rehabilitate addicts. Ford is a staff writer for the *Christian Science Monitor*, an international daily newspaper.

On a winter afternoon, Udi Aviaz strolls into Kadinsky's coffee shop just off one of Amsterdam's famed canals and asks to see the menu.

But the pages of the purple-ring binder do not list drinks. They list drugs.

Mr. Aviaz, an Israeli living in Holland, selects a joint of locally grown marijuana, orders a Coke, and sits down to listen to B.B. King while he gets high. "What I like about Holland is that the sense of paranoia is gone," he says. "I can totally enjoy smoking, and I feel quite safe."

Holland, which has allowed the possession of small amounts of marijuana, or cannabis, for the past 25 years, was once alone in its permissive stance. But more and more European countries are following its lead and turning their backs on Washington's war on drugs. The trend is bolstered by figures showing that Holland's radical approach has not led to greater drug use, and has improved addicts' health.

Drug consumption is generally far lower in Europe than in the U.S. Eighteen percent of Dutch people have smoked marijuana at least once, for example, compared with 33 percent of Americans.

Reprinted, with permission, from "Europe Shifts Out of Drug-War Mode," by Peter Ford, *Christian Science Monitor*, March 12, 2001.

Sending a Different Message

"Where the American slogan is 'Just Say No,' the European policy is 'Just Say Know,'" explains Danilo Ballotta, an expert with the Lisbon-based European Monitoring Center for Drugs and Drug Addiction, the European Union's (EU) drug agency. "Our policies are completely different, and our messages are completely different."

The Dutch government is growing less defensive about its pioneering focus on reducing the risks that go with taking drugs: While drug possession is technically against the law, the government has chosen not to prosecute over small-scale consumption and to go after wholesale dealers and producers instead.

Other countries are changing their focus, too. The Belgian government announced in February 2001 that it will formally decriminalize personal use of marijuana, and a similar bill is before the Luxembourg parliament. The Swiss parliament will soon debate a law permitting people to smoke cannabis, and in July 2001 a new Portuguese law comes into effect that will decriminalize the personal use of all drugs, hard and soft.

The British government announced recently it would draw up new guidelines for police, recommending that they do nothing when small quantities of cannabis are found; French authorities do not prosecute 95 percent of cannabis-possession cases, and in Spain, Italy, and most German regions the police turn a blind eye. Only in Sweden and Greece have authorities still fixed their goal on a drug-free society.

European drug officials insist that their policies do not mean they have surrendered to drugs.

Dutch police regularly cooperate with their Belgian, German, and French counterparts in seizing large quantities of cannabis and other illicit substances in operations to control roads and trains.

Instead of an all-out war on drugs, European governments are increasingly turning to what they call "harm reduction" policies. "We don't want to chase drug users," says Nicoline van der Arend, an adviser to the Dutch Minister of Justice. "If we don't arrest them and put them in prison, perhaps they will be willing to have treatment."

"We treat them as addicts, not as criminals. The fundamental point is that this is a public-health problem more than a law-and-order problem," argues Peter Pennekamp, director general of the Dutch Health Ministry. "If you are aware that risks are being taken, you can either ignore it, or do something to reduce the risks."

That approach has spurred the creation of needle-exchange programs throughout Western Europe, giving addicts clean syringes so as to lower the chances they will be infected with HIV or hepatitis. Germany and Spain have recently followed Holland's example and opened "shooting rooms," where drugs can be consumed under hygienic and supervised conditions. All 15 EU members run substitution programs, offering heroin addicts methadone instead. And

Dutch voluntary organizations take mobile pill-testing labs to rave parties, checking the quality of the Ecstasy often sold to dancers.

The Impact of European Policies

All European governments run widespread campaigns to persuade young people not to take drugs. They say this realism pays off. In Holland, for example, the number of cannabis users is about average for Europe, and the number of "problematic" hard-drug users is among the lowest on the Continent. Holland has the lowest overdose death rate in Europe, except for France. The Dutch are alone, however, in permitting coffee shops to sell as much as five grams of hashish or marijuana per customer.

This is a bid to keep young people who want to smoke marijuana out of hard-drug circles, which they might fall into if they frequented illegal dealers.

But the policy is full of ambiguities and paradoxes: Coffee shops may sell to customers, for example, but their suppliers are breaking the law. "We pay taxes on everything we sell," says Vijay Shamdas, the barman at Kadinsky's. "But they don't know what we bought or what it cost because they turn a blind eye."

Few of Holland's neighbors are expected to go as far as The Hague has gone. Belgium is going half-way, decriminalizing cannabis and boosting government funds for programs that educate young people to stay away from drugs, or help rehabilitate drug addicts. "Prevention is better than cure, and a cure is better than punishment," the ministries of Health and Justice said in a joint statement.

"We want to avoid making cannabis use seem normal, but we don't want to dramatize it either," said a government announcement. "We will put the emphasis on prevention, and the authorities should intervene only when consumption [of cannabis] gives rise to problems."

Portugal has taken a wider approach, decriminalizing the use of all drugs as part of a new public-health strategy to be launched in July 2001. There, says Mr. Ballotta, "decriminalization is a tool to improve the treatment option. You keep the user out of prison, so that you can try to start a treatment and rehabilitation process."

After years of vilification from neighboring governments for running a "narco-state," Dutch officials are quietly pleased to see their policies copied. "We say that our policy suits The Netherlands, that people should take the information here and fit it to their countries," says Mr. Pennekamp. "Slowly people are getting inspired."

CHAPTER 3

THE CONTROVERSY OVER MEDICAL MARIJUANA

THE MEDICAL MARIJUANA DEBATE: AN OVERVIEW

Elisabeth Frater

Despite federal laws prohibiting marijuana, in 1996, California and Arizona passed state initiatives legalizing marijuana for medical use by patients suffering from serious illnesses. These initiatives sparked a national debate over the medical use of marijuana, which Elisabeth Frater explores in the following selection. Frater explains that supporters of the initiatives believe marijuana has true health benefits, such as providing relief from pain and nausea when traditional medications prove ineffective. The federal government and anti-drug groups, on the other hand, maintain that medical marijuana initiatives are simply a tactic employed by legalization proponents to downplay the dangers of marijuana and promote complete legalization of the drug, she writes. Frater is an intern reporter for the *National Journal*.

A controversial assault on the nation's war on illegal drugs started in 1996, when a well-organized and well-funded coalition of drug law reformers and grass-roots activists put legalization of "medical marijuana" on the ballots in California and Arizona. Propelled by evidence that marijuana sometimes alleviates the symptoms or side effects suffered by some seriously ill people who do not respond to conventional medicine, the first two legalization measures proved enormously popular, winning 65 percent of the vote in Arizona and 56 percent in California.

Opposing Medical Marijuana Initiatives

Surprised by the measures' success, the Clinton Administration mobilized within days to develop a game plan aimed at defeating similar initiatives in other states and preventing the drive to legalize medical marijuana from expanding to cover all uses of marijuana. The government's aggressive response triggered a high-profile legal clash over whether "medical necessity" is a permissible justification for violating federal drug-possession laws. That dispute will be heard by the U.S. Supreme Court on March 28, 2001. [On May 14, 2001, the U.S.

Supreme Court ruled that California cannabis clubs may not distribute marijuana as a medical necessity.]

Gen. Barry McCaffrey, who was the Clinton Administration's drug czar in 1996, recalls: "My own solid judgment was that there were a . . . small number of people, a few hundred, who were determined to make the use of smoked marijuana more tolerated, legal, readily available. . . . They've got money, and they've got energy."

At McCaffrey's urging, representatives of the Justice Department, the Drug Enforcement Agency (DEA), the Office of National Drug Control Policy, and the state governments of California and Arizona met on Nov. 14, 1996, with anti-drug interest groups, including the Partnership for a Drug-Free America and Community Anti-Drug Coalitions of America. According to official notes from that session, the foes of medical marijuana lamented that they had been blindsided by "stealth legislation," and they characterized the organizers of the initiatives as "using the terminally ill as props."

James E. Copple, then-president of Community Anti-Drug Coalitions of America, argued at the meeting that the other 48 states needed to be protected from medical marijuana propaganda, and he described plans to spread a counter-message in seven states.

But Thomas Gede, then a special assistant attorney general of California, cautioned the group against taking more extreme measures, such as seizing medical marijuana or arresting those who distributed it. He said he feared potential government liability if ill people suffered or died because they could not receive the medical marijuana approved by their states. DEA officials chimed in to warn that the federal court system would "grind . . . to a halt" if it were flooded with relatively petty marijuana arrests.

Despite federal efforts to counter it, the medical marijuana cause continued to win resounding victories at the state level: By 2000, ballot initiatives legalizing the medical use of marijuana had easily passed in Alaska, Colorado, Nevada, Oregon, Maine, and Washington. Also in 2000, Hawaii's state Legislature became the first to approve medical marijuana.

The Cannabis Cooperatives

Yet, state-level medical marijuana measures have proven to be imperfect vehicles for their cause, because they don't specify how the marijuana can wend its way from growers or suppliers to patients without breaking federal law. Cooperatives have been created to dispense medical marijuana in various forms, but some, including the Oakland Cannabis Buyers' Cooperative in California, have been targeted by the federal lawsuit intended to shut them down.

In March 2001, the U.S. Supreme Court will hear arguments in *United States vs. Oakland Cannabis Buyers' Cooperative*, the federal government's lawsuit to stop what it considers to be the illegal sale and distribution of marijuana by California clubs and cooperatives.

The Oakland cooperative is under court order to stop dispensing marijuana while the case is pending. Now the cooperative dispenses only advice and good wishes. Jeffrey Jones, its executive director, says: "We are important to the social and beneficial atmosphere that these patients need, to keep on top of their condition and . . . not give up on their life—[unlike] the cold shoulder and the indifferent hand that the federal government has offered them."

The perceived threat posed by cannabis cooperatives is not that there are too many for the feds to suppress. According to the National Organization for the Reform of Marijuana Laws, there are only 30 to 40 such groups in the country. Instead, federal officials are acting out of the conviction, shared by anti-drug groups, that medical marijuana is dangerous in itself—and also is the stalking horse for efforts to legalize all marijuana use.

The Politics of Medical Marijuana

As Betty Sembler, founder of the Drug-Free America Foundation in St. Petersburg, Fla., puts it: "First of all, I don't call it medicinal marijuana, because there is no such thing. Marijuana is *medical excuse* marijuana. That's all it is. The pro-drug lobby is trying to use it to say it's a natural thing to do, to burn your lungs, ruin your mind. . . . It's just part of a marketing agenda."

Timothy Lynch, director of the criminal justice program for the libertarian Cato Institute, says, "Medical marijuana represents the first step in the direction of de-escalating the war" on drugs.

Still, given the evident public support for medical marijuana, why has the government continued to fight it? Eric E. Sterling, president of the Criminal Justice Policy Foundation, thinks one reason is that the issue creates a tug-of-war "between the conservative viewpoint of traditional values and those who reject traditional values." In his view, "The war on drugs is not only a policy matter, it is a crusade."

Congressional Republicans were among those pressuring federal drug fighters to combat medical marijuana. In October 1997, McCaffrey was summoned to testify before the House crime subcommittee chaired by then-Rep. Bill McCollum, R-Fla., who said he was worried about a possible medical marijuana initiative in his state and "the potential consequences of a shift in public policy toward marijuana legalization." Rep. Asa Hutchinson, R-Ark., sternly ordered McCaffrey "to be more engaged in the battle."

R. Keith Stroup, the founder and executive director of the National Organization for the Reform of Marijuana Laws, says that he thinks "the Republican [congressional] leadership some time ago chose to make its opposition to the medical use of marijuana a major plank in their anti-drug war. . . . " Stroup recalls that in 1981, McCollum and then-Rep. Newt Gingrich, R-Ga., co-sponsored a bill to allow the therapeutic use of marijuana in situations involving life-threatening illnesses.

"Yet," Stroup said, "years later, when the war on drugs is running strong and the Republicans are trying to take advantage of it, they actually led the charge against medical marijuana. Nothing had changed . . . except that the Republicans had taken a particular strategic position."

However, it was a Democratic Administration whose drug czar and Attorney General actually challenged the marijuana cooperatives.

Former drug czar McCaffrey denies that obliterating medical marijuana was a personal crusade for him and says that he considered it a trifling issue, compared with other narcotics problems. He adds that he viewed the medical marijuana conflict largely as a medical matter that should be decided in the "forum of science and medicine."

Looking to Science for Answers

Many anti-drug organizations agree with McCaffrey's view. For example, Howard Simon, spokesman for Partnership for a Drug-Free America, says: "Voters should not circumvent recognized scientific and medical processes by deciding what constitutes safe and effective medicine via the ballot box. Let's not politicize it. Let's not emotionalize it. . . . Let's let the scientists and researchers give us the answer—the same way the [Food and Drug Administration] would look at any other proposed medication."

In January 1997, McCaffrey commissioned the National Academy of Sciences' (NAS) Institute of Medicine to assess the potential health benefits and risks of marijuana and tetrahydrocannabinol (THC), the primary psychoactive ingredient in marijuana. Both sides found some support for their views in the NAS report, which was released in March 1999.

Pro-marijuana groups embraced the researchers' conclusion that "there are some limited circumstances in which we recommend smoking marijuana for medical uses." The report found that marijuana has "potential therapeutic value" when used for pain relief, control of chemotherapy-induced nausea, and appetite stimulation in AIDS patients.

The government latched onto another of the report's conclusions: "Although marijuana smoke delivers THC and other cannabinoids to the body, it also delivers harmful substances, including most of those found in tobacco smoke." The American Medical Association, which is reviewing its position, recommends "adequate and well-controlled studies of smoked marijuana" and urges the National Institutes of Health to develop smoke-free methods of administering marijuana to patients.

According to a March 1999 Gallup Poll, although 69 percent of American adults say they oppose the general decriminalization of marijuana, 73 percent favor making marijuana "legally available for doctors to prescribe in order to reduce pain and suffering."

Most observers doubt that the outcome of the medical marijuana case now before the Supreme Court will provide the final word on the larger controversy. Sterling predicts that public opinion will eventually force the federal government to "change its position, over the objections of DEA and the Justice Department."

Sterling concluded: "The American people understand that making marijuana available to sick people to relieve their conditions is nothing like legalizing marijuana for other kinds of uses. . . . [Medical marijuana] is not going to drive a stake into the heart of law enforcement, as some tend to exaggerate."

EXAMINING THE SCIENTIFIC RESEARCH ON MEDICAL MARIJUANA

The Institute of Medicine

The Institute of Medicine (IOM), a division of the National Academy of Sciences, provides the federal government with information and advice on policy matters pertaining to public health. In January 1997, the White House Office of National Drug Control Policy asked the IOM to review the scientific evidence on the potential health benefits and risks of marijuana. The following excerpt from the institute's report, *Marijuana and Medicine: Assessing the Science Base*, summarizes the IOM's conclusions and recommendations. According to the IOM, research shows that marijuana has potential therapeutic value, especially in the relief of pain, control of nausea, and stimulation of appetite. However, the IOM notes, marijuana would only be effective as medicine for a limited number of patients. Furthermore, because of the chronic health risks associated with inhaling smoke, the IOM recommends only short-term use of smoked marijuana and advocates further research into the development of nonsmoked forms of marijuana's active ingredients.

Public opinion on the medical value of marijuana has been sharply divided. Some dismiss medical marijuana as a hoax that exploits our natural compassion for the sick; others claim it is a uniquely soothing medicine that has been withheld from patients through regulations based on false claims. Proponents of both views cite "scientific evidence" to support their views and have expressed those views at the ballot box in recent state elections. In January 1997, the White House Office of National Drug Control Policy (ONDCP) asked the Institute of Medicine (IOM) to conduct a review of the scientific evidence to assess the potential health benefits and risks of marijuana and its constituent cannabinoids. That review began in August 1997 and culminates with this report.

The ONDCP request came in the wake of state "medical marijuana" initiatives. In November 1996, voters in California and Arizona

Reprinted from The Institute of Medicine, "Executive Summary," *Marijuana and Medicine: Assessing the Science Base.* Copyright © 1999 The National Academy of Sciences. Used by permission of National Academy Press.

passed referenda designed to permit the use of marijuana as medicine. Although Arizona's referendum was invalidated five months later, the referenda galvanized a national response. In November 1998, voters in six states (Alaska, Arizona, Colorado, Nevada, Oregon, and Washington) passed ballot initiatives in support of medical marijuana. (The Colorado vote will not count, however, because after the vote was taken a court ruling determined there had not been enough valid signatures to place the initiative on the ballot.)

Evaluating the Evidence

Can marijuana relieve health problems? Is it safe for medical use? Those straightforward questions are embedded in a web of social concerns, most of which lie outside the scope of this report. Controversies concerning the nonmedical use of marijuana spill over into the medical marijuana debate and obscure the real state of scientific knowledge. In contrast with the many disagreements bearing on social issues, the study team found substantial consensus among experts in the relevant disciplines on the scientific evidence about potential medical uses of marijuana.

This report summarizes and analyzes what is known about the medical use of marijuana; it emphasizes evidence-based medicine (derived from knowledge and experience informed by rigorous scientific analysis), as opposed to belief-based medicine (derived from judgment, intuition, and beliefs untested by rigorous science).

Throughout this report, *marijuana* refers to unpurified plant substances, including leaves or flower tops whether consumed by ingestion or smoking. References to the "effects of marijuana" should be understood to include the composite effects of its various components; that is, the effects of tetrahydrocannabinol (THC), which is the primary psychoactive ingredient in marijuana, are included among its effects, but not all the effects of marijuana are necessarily due to THC. *Cannabinoids* are the group of compounds related to THC, whether found in the marijuana plant, in animals, or synthesized in chemistry laboratories.

Three focal concerns in evaluating the medical use of marijuana are:
1. Evaluation of the effects of isolated cannabinoids;
2. Evaluation of the risks associated with the medical use of marijuana; and
3. Evaluation of the use of smoked marijuana.

Studying Cannabinoid Biology

Much has been learned since the 1982 IOM report *Marijuana and Health*. Although it was clear then that most of the effects of marijuana were due to its actions on the brain, there was little information about how THC acted on brain cells (neurons), which cells were affected by THC, or even what general areas of the brain were most affected by

THC. In addition, too little was known about cannabinoid physiology to offer any scientific insights into the harmful or therapeutic effects of marijuana. That all changed with the identification and characterization of cannabinoid receptors in the 1980s and 1990s. During the past 16 years, science has advanced greatly and can tell us much more about the potential medical benefits of cannabinoids.

Conclusion: At this point, our knowledge about the biology of marijuana and cannabinoids allows us to make some general conclusions:

- Cannabinoids likely have a natural role in pain modulation, control of movement, and memory.
- The natural role of cannabinoids in immune systems is likely multi-faceted and remains unclear.
- The brain develops tolerance to cannabinoids.
- Animal research demonstrates the potential for dependence, but this potential is observed under a narrower range of conditions than with benzodiazepines, opiates, cocaine, or nicotine.
- Withdrawal symptoms can be observed in animals but appear to be mild compared to opiates or benzodiazepines, such as diazepam (Valium).

Conclusion: The different cannabinoid receptor types found in the body appear to play different roles in normal human physiology. In addition, some effects of cannabinoids appear to be independent of those receptors. The variety of mechanisms through which cannabinoids can influence human physiology underlies the variety of potential therapeutic uses for drugs that might act selectively on different cannabinoid systems.

Recommendation 1: Research should continue into the physiological effects of synthetic and plant-derived cannabinoids and the natural function of cannabinoids found in the body. Because different cannabinoids appear to have different effects, cannabinoid research should include, but not be restricted to, effects attributable to THC alone.

The Efficacy of Cannabinoid Drugs

The accumulated data indicate a potential therapeutic value for cannabinoid drugs, particularly for symptoms such as pain relief, control of nausea and vomiting, and appetite stimulation. The therapeutic effects of cannabinoids are best established for THC, which is generally one of the two most abundant of the cannabinoids in marijuana. (Cannabidiol is generally the other most abundant cannabinoid.)

The effects of cannabinoids on the symptoms studied are generally modest, and in most cases there are more effective medications. However, people vary in their responses to medications, and there will likely always be a subpopulation of patients who do not respond well to other medications. The combination of cannabinoid drug effects (anxiety reduction, appetite stimulation, nausea reduction, and pain relief) suggests that cannabinoids would be moderately well suited for particular conditions, such as chemotherapy-induced nausea and vomiting and AIDS wasting.

Defined substances, such as purified cannabinoid compounds, are preferable to plant products, which are of variable and uncertain composition. Use of defined cannabinoids permits a more precise evaluation of their effects, whether in combination or alone. Medications that can maximize the desired effects of cannabinoids and minimize the undesired effects can very likely be identified.

Although most scientists who study cannabinoids agree that the pathways to cannabinoid drug development are clearly marked, there is no guarantee that the fruits of scientific research will be made available to the public for medical use. Cannabinoid-based drugs will only become available if public investment in cannabinoid drug research is sustained and if there is enough incentive for private enterprise to develop and market such drugs.

Conclusion: Scientific data indicate the potential therapeutic value of cannabinoid drugs, primarily THC, for pain relief, control of nausea and vomiting, and appetite stimulation; smoked marijuana, however, is a crude THC delivery system that also delivers harmful substances.

Recommendation 2: Clinical trials of cannabinoid drugs for symptom management should be conducted with the goal of developing rapid-onset, reliable, and safe delivery systems.

Psychological Effects

The psychological effects of THC and similar cannabinoids pose three issues for the therapeutic use of cannabinoid drugs. First, for some patients—particularly older patients with no previous marijuana experience—the psychological effects are disturbing. Those patients report experiencing unpleasant feelings and disorientation after being treated with THC, generally more severe for oral THC than for smoked marijuana. Second, for conditions such as movement disorders or nausea, in which anxiety exacerbates the symptoms, the antianxiety effects of cannabinoid drugs can influence symptoms indirectly. This can be beneficial or can create false impressions of the drug effect. Third, for cases in which symptoms are multifaceted, the combination of THC effects might provide a form of adjunctive therapy; for example, AIDS wasting patients would likely benefit from a medication that simultaneously reduces anxiety, pain, and nausea while stimulating appetite.

Conclusion: The psychological effects of cannabinoids, such as anxiety reduction, sedation, and euphoria, can influence their potential therapeutic value. Those effects are potentially undesirable for certain patients and situations and beneficial for others. In addition, psychological effects can complicate the interpretation of other aspects of the drug's effect.

Recommendation 3: Psychological effects of cannabinoids such as anxiety reduction and sedation, which can influence medical benefits, should be evaluated in clinical trials.

Physiological Risks

Marijuana is not a completely benign substance. It is a powerful drug with a variety of effects. However, except for the harms associated with smoking, the adverse effects of marijuana use are within the range of effects tolerated for other medications. The harmful effects to individuals from the perspective of possible medical use of marijuana are not necessarily the same as the harmful physical effects of drug abuse. When interpreting studies purporting to show the harmful effects of marijuana, it is important to keep in mind that the majority of those studies are based on *smoked* marijuana, and cannabinoid effects cannot be separated from the effects of inhaling smoke from burning plant material and contaminants.

For most people the primary adverse effect of *acute* marijuana use is diminished psychomotor performance. It is, therefore, inadvisable to operate any vehicle or potentially dangerous equipment while under the influence of marijuana, THC, or any cannabinoid drug with comparable effects. In addition, a minority of marijuana users experience dysphoria, or unpleasant feelings. Finally, the short-term immunosuppressive effects are not well established but, if they exist, are not likely great enough to preclude a legitimate medical use.

The *chronic* effects of marijuana are of greater concern for medical use and fall into two categories: the effects of chronic smoking and the effects of THC. Marijuana smoking is associated with abnormalities of cells lining the human respiratory tract. Marijuana smoke, like tobacco smoke, is associated with increased risk of cancer, lung damage, and poor pregnancy outcomes. Although cellular, genetic, and human studies all suggest that marijuana smoke is an important risk factor for the development of respiratory cancer, proof that habitual marijuana smoking does or does not cause cancer awaits the results of well-designed studies.

Conclusion: Numerous studies suggest that marijuana smoke is an important risk factor in the development of respiratory disease.

Recommendation 4: Studies to define the individual health risks of smoking marijuana should be conducted, particularly among populations in which marijuana use is prevalent.

A second concern associated with chronic marijuana use is dependence on the psychoactive effects of THC. Although few marijuana users develop dependence, some do. Risk factors for marijuana dependence are similar to those for other forms of substance abuse. In particular, anti-social personality and conduct disorders are closely associated with substance abuse.

Conclusion: A distinctive marijuana withdrawal syndrome has been identified, but it is mild and short lived. The syndrome includes restlessness, irritability, mild agitation, insomnia, sleep disturbance, nausea, and cramping.

A "Gateway" Drug?

Patterns in progression of drug use from adolescence to adulthood are strikingly regular. Because it is the most widely used illicit drug, marijuana is predictably the first illicit drug most people encounter. Not surprisingly, most users of other illicit drugs have used marijuana first. In fact, most drug users begin with alcohol and nicotine before marijuana—usually before they are of legal age.

In the sense that marijuana use typically precedes rather than follows initiation of other illicit drug use, it is indeed a "gateway" drug. But because underage smoking and alcohol use typically precede marijuana use, marijuana is not the most common, and is rarely the first, "gateway" to illicit drug use. There is no conclusive evidence that the drug effects of marijuana are causally linked to the subsequent abuse of other illicit drugs. An important caution is that data on drug use progression cannot be assumed to apply to the use of drugs for medical purposes. It does not follow from those data that if marijuana were available by prescription for medical use, the pattern of drug use would remain the same as seen in illicit use.

Finally, there is a broad social concern that sanctioning the medical use of marijuana might increase its use among the general population. At this point there are no convincing data to support this concern. The existing data are consistent with the idea that this would not be a problem if the medical use of marijuana were as closely regulated as other medications with abuse potential.

Conclusion: Present data on drug use progression neither support nor refute the suggestion that medical availability would increase drug abuse. However, this question is beyond the issues normally considered for medical uses of drugs and should not be a factor in evaluating the therapeutic potential of marijuana or cannabinoids.

Smoking Marijuana

Because of the health risks associated with smoking, smoked marijuana should generally not be recommended for long-term medical use. Nonetheless, for certain patients, such as the terminally ill or those with debilitating symptoms, the long-term risks are not of great concern. Further, despite the legal, social, and health problems associated with smoking marijuana, it is widely used by certain patient groups.

Recommendation 5: Clinical trials of marijuana use for medical purposes should be conducted under the following limited circumstances: trials should involve only short-term marijuana use (less than six months), should be conducted in patients with conditions for which there is reasonable expectation of efficacy, should be approved by institutional review boards, and should collect data about efficacy.

The goal of clinical trials of smoked marijuana would not be to develop marijuana as a licensed drug but rather to serve as a first step toward the possible development of nonsmoked rapid-onset cannabinoid delivery systems. However, it will likely be many years before a safe and effective cannabinoid delivery system, such as an inhaler, is available for patients. In the meantime there are patients with debilitating symptoms for whom smoked marijuana might provide relief. The use of smoked marijuana for those patients should weigh both the expected efficacy of marijuana and ethical issues in patient care, including providing information about the known and suspected risks of smoked marijuana use.

Recommendation 6: Short-term use of smoked marijuana (less than six months) for patients with debilitating symptoms (such as intractable pain or vomiting) must meet the following conditions:

- failure of all approved medications to provide relief has been documented,
- the symptoms can reasonably be expected to be relieved by rapid-onset cannabinoid drugs,
- such treatment is administered under medical supervision in a manner that allows for assessment of treatment effectiveness, and
- involves an oversight strategy comparable to an institutional review board process that could provide guidance within 24 hours of a submission by a physician to provide marijuana to a patient for a specified use.

Until a nonsmoked rapid-onset cannabinoid drug delivery system becomes available, we acknowledge that there is no clear alternative for people suffering from *chronic* conditions that might be relieved by smoking marijuana, such as pain or AIDS wasting. One possible approach is to treat patients as *n*-of-1 clinical trials (single-patient trials), in which patients are fully informed of their status as experimental subjects using a harmful drug delivery system and in which their condition is closely monitored and documented under medical supervision, thereby increasing the knowledge base of the risks and benefits of marijuana use under such conditions.

THE POTENTIAL MEDICAL BENEFITS OF MARIJUANA

Economist

The editors of the *Economist*, a British news magazine, review some of the possible medical uses for marijuana in the following selection. According to the *Economist*, smoking marijuana appears to alleviate the symptoms of glaucoma and multiple sclerosis, suppress the nausea resulting from chemotherapy, and stimulate the appetites of AIDS patients. The editors note that some alternative drug therapies are available for these conditions, but in many cases smoking marijuana is far less expensive than the alternatives. Although marijuana's active ingredient is also produced in the form of capsules, the editors maintain that smoking marijuana gives patients greater control over the dosage they receive.

"There is not a shred of scientific evidence . . . that smoked marijuana is useful or needed." Thus spake Barry McCaffrey, a retired army general and Gulf-war hero, in his role as commander-in-chief of the Clinton administration's War on Drugs. The National Institutes of Health (NIH) begs cautiously to differ. An NIH report issued on August 8, 1997, said that eight experts whom it had convened earlier in 1997 expressed "varying degrees of enthusiasm" about whether the dreaded weed had true medical value and, if it had, whether it did things that other drugs, less frowned upon by officialdom, could not. William Beaver of Georgetown University, who chaired the original workshop, said that "for at least some potential indications marijuana looks promising enough to recommend that there be new controlled studies."

Those who advocate marijuana as a medicine usually have four potential uses in mind: to control glaucoma, to suppress the nausea induced by anti-cancer drugs, to relieve the pain of multiple sclerosis, and to stimulate the appetites of those with AIDS.

The Benefits of Smoking Marijuana

In the case of glaucoma it is widely accepted that the elevated pressure in the eyeball that damages the optic nerve falls when marijuana is smoked. That is why, until 1991, America's Food and Drug Administration (FDA) permitted ophthalmologists to prescribe the weed to patients for whom other treatments had failed. Since then, new glaucoma drugs have been produced. These act at different points in the biochemical pathway that causes eyes to produce too much fluid. However, no approved drug actually makes the eyes' drainage system more efficient. If marijuana improves the outflow (which is possible, but not yet known) it would be a valuable addition to current therapies.

Marijuana is also of undoubted benefit in suppressing the nausea suffered by many people on anti-cancer chemotherapy. The argument here is whether it is necessary to smoke the stuff for the full benefits to emerge. This is because a capsule version of marijuana's active ingredient, delta-9-tetrahydrocannabinol, or THC, has been passed through the regulatory process for use in these circumstances.

Despite that, none of the NIH's experts deemed smoked marijuana to be by definition a superfluous adjunct to chemotherapy. Unlike oral THC, its vapour is easily absorbed and acts quickly. It may also contain as yet unidentified substances that help THC's action. And, unlike both the THC capsules and other legal nausea suppressors which work in different ways, reefers allow users to fine-tune the dose for themselves. Chemotherapy powerfully reminds cancer patients of their life-threatening illness. Because marijuana cigarettes are under their control, they tend to ease their feelings of helplessness.

In the case of multiple sclerosis (MS), marijuana brings relief that other painkillers do not seem to manage. Many of those who suffer from this disease have burning sensations in their limbs, particularly at night. These sensations are probably caused both by the disorder's destruction of the protective fatty coating around nerve cells and the damage it does to the brain.

Conventional analgesics can do little to ease this burning sensation—which seems to be similar to the phantom pain often suffered by amputees—but some sufferers say that a joint at bedtime makes the difference between their sleeping and not doing so. What study there has been of marijuana for MS—and it is not much—suggests they could be right.

The fourth use—marijuana's well-known ability to stimulate the appetite—is particularly significant in the treatment of AIDS. Again, smoking appears to be better than taking THC in capsule form. The pure form of the drug is poorly absorbed by many of the afflicted and, besides, often makes people so high that they never get around to eating. The loss of lean-muscle mass that occurs as patients waste away to shadows of their former selves is an ominous predictor of their impending deaths.

The best alternative to smoked pot for appetite stimulation is human growth hormone, which has been found both to restore lean tissue to emaciated AIDS patients and to improve their chances of survival. The catch is that—at $36,000 for a year's supply—it is pro-hibitively expensive (marijuana treatment for the same period costs a mere $500). The other readily available option is megestrol acetate, a synthetic female hormone which is somewhat cheaper. Unfortunately, studies have shown that it does not improve survival—probably because the weight gain it produces, instead of being mus-cle, is mainly fat.

All this would seem to make smoked marijuana the medicine of choice for helping the HIV-positive to gain the right kind of weight. Indeed, one AIDS patient testified to the workshop that it had enabled him to regain 40lbs (around 20kg), and that by using it only at night he had been able to keep that weight on for four years while working full-time as a newsletter editor.

Some studies done before the AIDS epidemic found, however, that marijuana dampens the immune system. Something that depresses their immune systems is the last thing that AIDS patients need. But these studies were only preliminary (others came to the opposite con-clusion) and they were done without the benefit of modern tech-niques for assessing immune-system damage. Unfortunately, they have not been repeated—which outlines one of the greatest difficul-ties in the effort to assess marijuana's value as a medical drug: doing trials to find out the truth.

Don't Ask, Don't Tell

A team of AIDS researchers, led by Donald Abrams of the University of California, San Francisco, planned a patient study aimed at resolving the immunity issue in 1992, but it was unable to get the marijuana that would have made the trial possible. The federal government is the only legal source of the drug for research purposes in America, and sci-entists cannot obtain it without the blessing of the NIH. In this case, the NIH stipulated that the proposal would first have to be given a suf-ficiently high score by an independent panel of scientific reviewers. But when the panelists received it, they refused to review it.

Their reasons for refusing are not entirely clear. Nor is it clear whether, assuming that such a study were carried out, and that it found marijuana to be an effective medicine, official approval for its use would then be forthcoming. [On September 18, 1997, the National Institute of Drug Abuse authorized the use of marijuana, under strict guidelines, for research on AIDS wasting syndrome.] America's food and drug law does not say that a drug has to be better than its com-petitors for a given purpose to be licensed. It has only to be better than a placebo. Nonetheless, Robert Temple, an FDA official, once said that his agency could be forced to withhold approval of smoked marijuana, despite this aspect of the law. Some drugs are known to induce paranoia through chemical action. Marijuana, it seems, can do it through political action instead.

MEDICAL MARIJUANA SHOULD NOT BE LEGALIZED

Bob Barr

In the following selection, Bob Barr argues that marijuana is a dangerous drug that should not be legalized for any reason. According to Barr, the campaign to legalize marijuana for medical purposes is simply a tactic employed by marijuana advocates to make marijuana and other drugs widely and legally available. No reputable studies have proven that smoking marijuana has any therapeutic value, he claims. However, Barr asserts, research has revealed marijuana's threat to public health: Marijuana contains carcinogens, impairs memory, and leads to use of other drugs. Furthermore, he maintains, the cost of accidents caused by people under the influence of marijuana in the workplace and on the roadways is substantial. Barr is a U.S. representative from the seventh district of Georgia who serves on the House Judiciary Committee.

In 1988, as the Reagan presidency and its successful "Just Say No" campaign were coming to a close, drug legalization advocates decided it was time for a change in tactics. With drug abuse rates actually dropping for the first time since the drug revolution began, and a White House strongly committed to fighting mind-altering drugs, the legalization movement faced a choice: become irrelevant, or camouflage its true goals in order to move its agenda forward. The movement chose for its disguise "Medical" marijuana.

The Legalization Strategy

As University of California at Los Angeles (UCLA) Public Policy Professor Mark Kleiman told the *New York Times* in June 1999, "[m]edical marijuana was chosen as a wedge issue several years ago by people who wanted to move drug policy in a softer direction."

In other words, the true aim of medicinal marijuana advocates is not to put drugs in the hands of doctors and pharmacists. Rather, the goal is to make marijuana and other drugs widely and legally available. To them, the medicinal-use argument is simply a contrived

From "Marijuana Should Not Be Legalized, Under Any Pretense," by Bob Barr, *Commonwealth,* June 1999.

means to an end, using terminally ill patients as pawns in a cynical political game.

From a purely political standpoint, the medicinal strategy has worked rather well for the legalizers. Backed by a handful of wealthy patrons like [international investor and philanthropist] George Soros, in a few short years legalization advocates have transformed themselves from socially unacceptable pariahs into the darlings of the national media. News reports on marijuana protestors at rallies became magically changed—with a speed that would make Cinderella green with envy—into stories about a repressive government denying "life-saving" drugs to "patients."

Putting the intellectual dishonesty of the legalization movement aside for a moment, let's take a look at the medicinal use argument on its own merits, or lack thereof.

Tetrahydrocannabinol (THC), the active ingredient in smoked marijuana, has been a legal prescription drug (marinol) available in the United States since 1984. For over a decade, physicians have been able to prescribe the active ingredient in marijuana. However, they rarely do, because other remedies—including drugs as well as medically-supervised pain management techniques—provide its therapeutic qualities more effectively. No reputable study has arrived at the conclusion that smoked marijuana has any therapeutic value sufficient to justify its medicinal use.

The Dangers of Marijuana

Not only is there no real proof that marijuana has any significant medicinal value, there is voluminous evidence that it is demonstrably harmful; if not deadly. For example, marijuana smoke contains roughly 30 times as many carcinogens as cigarette smoke. It is also dangerously addictive. Nationally, an estimated 100,000 individuals are in treatment for marijuana use.

Furthermore, inhalation of marijuana smoke depresses the immune system. This makes it likely that allowing its use by those with weak immune systems, such as Acquired Immune Deficiency Syndrome (AIDS) patients, would be highly questionable at best, and harmful at worst. Surely, well-informed observers would condemn a movement that fills the terminally ill with false hope, and encourages patients already vulnerable to pulmonary infections and tumors like Kaposi's sarcoma, to put a deadly substance in their lungs.

Moreover, marijuana use adversely affects the user's memory, a fact patently obvious in debates involving heavy marijuana users.

Marijuana use poses an even greater danger from a sociological standpoint than it does to the health of individuals who smoke it. Numerous studies have indicated marijuana use leads to abuse of other drugs like heroin, d-Lysergic Acid Diethylamide (LSD), and cocaine. Using data compiled by the Centers for Disease Control, researchers at Columbia University—hardly a bastion of conservative thought—concluded that children who drank, smoked cigarettes, or used marijuana at least once in the past month, were 16 times as likely to use another drug like cocaine, heroin, or LSD.

At the workplace, marijuana is a proven cause of absenteeism, accidents, and increased insurance claims. Estimates put the annual cost of on the job drug use at more than $100 billion per year.

On America's roads, marijuana poses a threat to all of us. Unlike alcohol, it is difficult to use roadside tests to determine the extent to which a driver is under the influence of marijuana, and there is practically no way for law enforcement to determine to what degree a particular driver's perception is altered by the drug, though by definition perception is altered (marijuana is a *mind-altering drug* for that reason). A recent study of reckless drivers found that 45% of those drivers not under the influence of alcohol tested positive for marijuana.

California has made national headlines by embarking on an obsessive campaign to eradicate cigarette smoking from public places. Ironically, in the same period, the state voted in favor of widely distributing a substance 30 times deadlier. What an imminently logical approach. What's next? Legalizing DDT and banning fly-swatters?

The Effects of Medicinal Legalization

Proponents of allowing doctors to dispense marijuana frequently make the simplistic, but media-friendly argument that doctors, not the government, should decide what drugs to prescribe. Accepting this premise, why have an FDA approval process at all? Why not just return to the 19th century, when "doctors" could prescribe any remedy—from powdered rhinoceros horn to sugar water in medicine bottles—that they personally felt was efficacious? Who needs science? Why not just ignore science, shut down the FDA, get rid of pharmacists, and stock pharmacy shelves by voter referendum?

Where else would medicinal legalization lead us? Undoubtedly, high school students—backed by the American Civil Liberties Union (ACLU)—would begin filing and winning lawsuits for permission to smoke their "medicine" in class, under a perverse interpretation of the equal protection clause of the Constitution. Others, from prisoners to bus drivers, would assuredly do the same.

Medicinal use would create a nightmare for employers. Accidents would increase, and employers could no longer test workers for drug use, for fear of winding up in court. Adding insult to injury, companies would be forced to pay for workers to get stoned on the job by including marijuana "treatment" in health plans. Everyone who drives a car would also be forced to foot the bill for this folly, in the form of increased accidents and higher insurance rates.

The bottom line is that legalization advocates don't care about any of these things. They are motivated either by a simple desire to smoke dope because it makes them feel good, or a misguided political philosophy that tells them legalizing drugs would end crime with one magical puff of smoke.

Unfortunately, citizens of several states have been all too eager to buy the snake oil legalizers are selling, because it is tantalizingly packaged in fake compassion and false hope for the sick. Hopefully, voters in other states will take the time to carefully consider the facts before they make an ill-formed decision to follow California's example.

THE FEDERAL GOVERNMENT SHOULD NOT INTERFERE WITH STATE MEDICAL MARIJUANA LAWS

Gary Newkirk

If the voting citizens of a state decide that they approve of the medical use of marijuana, the federal government should not interfere, argues Gary Newkirk in the following selection. Rather than deny medical marijuana to those patients for whom it may be beneficial, Newkirk asserts, the federal government should devise a policy that allows for the regulated and controlled use of the drug. For instance, he suggests, the federal government could oversee the cultivation and distribution of medical marijuana while sponsoring scientific research into marijuana's effectiveness. Newkirk is a clinical professor in the department of family practice at the University of Washington School of Medicine in Seattle and the medical editor of *Modern Medicine*, a monthly magazine for the healthcare industry.

On November 3, 1998, the voters of Washington State took the plunge and passed legislation legalizing the use of medicinal marijuana. The new law would allow the personal cultivation and use of smoked marijuana for certain chronic or terminal medical conditions when prescribed by a physician. The federal government, however, still classifies the personal use of smoked marijuana as a violation of federal statutes controlling the use of Schedule 1 drugs—that is, those drugs with high addiction potential and no demonstrated medicinal use. In fact, physicians and patients using this medication put themselves at potential risk for violation of federal statutes, including arrest and prosecution.

A Special Request

Recently, I became aware of a patient with a special request. She was diagnosed with bronchogenic lung cancer 2 years ago. The tumor was inoperable but responded to radiotherapy. At the present time, the tumor has stabilized in size but the patient is troubled by ongoing

Reprinted, with permission, from "It's Just a Weed," *Modern Medicine*, vol. 67, issue 6, p9, 2p, June 1999. Copyright © 2001 Advanstar Communications Inc. Advanstar Communications Inc. retains all rights to this material.

anorexia and insidious weight loss. Everything was tried to help improve this patient's nutritional status, including trials of anabolic steroids and Marinol (dronabinol), a drug that contains one of the active ingredients in marijuana. Unfortunately, none of these strategies provided anything but temporary abatement of weight loss. Although this patient was a heavy smoker, she quit smoking when the diagnosis of lung cancer was made. The thought of smoking "dope" was at first very threatening to her, both because it was smoking again and because it was marijuana.

Eventually, a supply of "weed" was procured and she tried it on her own. Smoking "pot" three or four times per day has allowed the patient to maintain her weight. However, the therapy has been very expensive, and the patient asked if there was a way to get marijuana plants or seeds legally so that she can maintain her weight. Unfortunately, I found that as I delved further into this issue, getting more information did not clarify matters at all.

The Voters Speak?

To begin with, there is a real fundamental problem between the role and responsibilities of the federal government and those of the states. It is obvious that even though a state's voting citizens want something and prevail through the electoral process, it doesn't mean they are going to get it. Soon after the legislation was passed regarding the use of medicinal marijuana, numerous branches of the federal government—from the President and the Attorney General to the director of the Office of National Drug Control Policy—exerted its condemnation by various threats, disclaimers, and warnings. Attorney General Janet Reno, for example, announced that physicians who prescribed the drug could lose the privilege of writing prescriptions, be excluded from Medicare and Medicaid reimbursement, and even be prosecuted for a federal crime.

Am I just getting paranoid, or is the federal government getting back in the office again? Arguments against the use of medicinal marijuana run the gamut from concerns over making marijuana available "on every street corner" (Isn't it already?) to encouraging Americans to give up their lettuce and tomato gardens in favor of growing marijuana. Another argument states that there are available and satisfactory alternatives to the use of marijuana. Indeed there are, but let us recall that the legitimate use of morphine and other narcotics has not led to a proliferation of opium poppy gardens in Grandma's backyard either!

The suffering experienced by those with chronic and/or terminal disease is immeasurable, and not all drugs work equally well for all patients. Indeed, there may be adequate choices for the treatment of uncomplicated pain, but the therapeutic index for most such medications is extremely narrow and they are not tolerated by everyone. Two of the most elusive symptoms cancer patients suffer include dysphoria [a state of anxiety, depression, and restlessness] and anorexia, for which little can be done. If there is even a remote chance that the compounds available in the smoked version of marijuana can help, then that possibility should be pursued with at least as much clinical fervor and research as the search that led to identification of effective drugs for the treatment of erectile dysfunction.

It is estimated that smoking native marijuana delivers nearly 400 different bioactive compounds. At least from an intuitive perspective, therefore, it is not surprising that the oral, purified, synthetic version of one of marijuana's major ingredients may not demonstrate the same benefits as the native plant when smoked. Indeed, the discovery of receptors in the central nervous system for cannabinoid compounds must certainly tantalize even the staunchest skeptic that more research is necessary. We already live in an age when we inhale or otherwise snort medications for a variety of medical conditions, from pain control, to migraine, to asthma, to osteoporosis. Smoking marijuana delivers a very rapid dose of these various compounds, and it may be that the interaction of the various components as well as the delivery through the respiratory system accounts for the perception that smoked marijuana has unique effects.

Clearly, like most drugs, particularly when not yet refined and quantified, smoked marijuana likely will have untoward effects, but in the context of managing terminal symptoms, the concept of "benefit to risk" takes on a whole new meaning. Given the immeasurable human suffering experienced by a large portion of the population near the end of life, surely we can muster enough funding and unbiased intellectual pursuit to thoroughly investigate the use and effectiveness of marijuana as a valid medicinal agent. The federal government's real role here is in basic research.

And just so that no one entity feels picked on, I am equally suspicious of those who claim that smoking marijuana is a cure for everything. The various state statutes regarding medicinal marijuana have bizarre applications. In most instances, the new laws allow patients to grow their own supply "for personal consumption." Who in the world thought that one up? I envision a million little legal "pot gardens" throughout the country; should we actually expect that the crop wouldn't somehow be misused? No wonder the federal government is concerned. Likewise, we can fire up the old prohibition stills! Should patients grow their own opium poppies?

The Real Role of the Government

Perhaps the appropriate role for the federal government would be to oversee the growing and cultivation of the medicinal marijuana to help control its distribution and consistency in clinical settings where benefits outweigh the risks. Rather than having a power showdown over this issue, which traps patients and providers in the crossfire, why don't the federal government and states work together to provide a medicinal marijuana policy that can not only provide potential relief to citizens in desperate need, but at the same time stage ongoing research regarding its effectiveness and applicability?

Who among us knows for sure that at the end of our life we will not benefit from the use of medicinal marijuana? As for my patient, I am not really sure what to tell her, and that is the real crime, since the marijuana issue has been raging on and on for years—under funded and overpoliticized. Let's make some changes right now. Marijuana is currently a Schedule 1 drug, considered to be potentially addictive and with no current medical use. Marijuana needs to be reclassified as a Schedule 2 drug, "potentially addictive but with some accepted medical use," and studied to the hilt by the same impartial science that has brought this country to the forefront in medicine. I am quite confident that if the truly active and effective ingredients in smoked marijuana are identified, that some good, enterprising pharmaceutical company will rise to the occasion and produce a reliable and available product.

Please, let's quit fooling around. People are suffering! In the meantime, leave the "practice of medicine" to those of us who practice medicine.

STATE MEDICAL MARIJUANA LAWS THREATEN THE PUBLIC HEALTH

James R. McDonough

In the following selection, James R. McDonough, director of the Florida Office of Drug Control, argues that smoking marijuana is hazardous to the public health and should remain illegal. According to the author, state laws that permit the smoking of marijuana for medical purposes circumvent the protection of the public health by bypassing the approval process of the Federal Drug Administration. These state laws are problematic because they do not regulate the purity and dosage of smoked marijuana, he explains, and they often do not specify the medical conditions for which it may be prescribed. The federal government is correct in its attempts to interfere with these state laws, McDonough concludes, especially because marijuana's medical benefits have yet to be proven, while the health risks of inhaling marijuana smoke are well documented.

While it has long been clear that chemical compounds found in the marijuana plant offer potential for medical use, smoking the raw plant is a method of delivery supported neither by law nor recent scientific evidence. The Food and Drug Administration's approval process, which seeks to ensure the purity of chemical compounds in legitimate drugs, sets the standard for medical validation of prescription drugs as safe and effective. Diametrically opposed to this long-standing safeguard of medical science is the recent spate of state election ballots that have advocated the use of a smoked plant—the marijuana leaf—for "treating" an unspecified number of ailments. It is a tribute to the power of political activism that popular vote has displaced objective science in advancing what would be the only smoked drug in America under the guise of good medicine.

Two recent studies of the potential medical utility of marijuana advocate development of a non-smoked, rapid onset delivery system of the cannabis compounds. But state ballot initiatives that seek legalization of smoking marijuana as medicine threaten to circumvent credible research. Advocates for smoking marijuana appear to want to

From James R. McDonough, "Marijuana on the Ballot," *Policy Review*, April/May 2000, published by *The Heritage Foundation*. Used with permission.

move ahead at all costs, irrespective of dangers to the user. They make a well-financed, emotional appeal to the voting public claiming that what they demand is humane, useful, and safe. Although they rely largely on anecdote to document their claims, they seize upon partial statements that purport to validate their assertions. At the same time, these partisans—described by Chris Wren, the highly respected journalist for the *New York Times*, as a small coalition of libertarians, liberals, humanitarians, and hedonists—reject the main conclusions of medical science: that there is little future in smoked marijuana as a medically approved medication.

A Dearth of Scientific Support

Compounds found in marijuana may have medical potential, but science does not support smoking the plant in its crude form as an appropriate delivery system. An exploration of two comprehensive inquiries into the medical potential of marijuana indicates the following:

- Science has identified only the potential medical benefit of chemical compounds, such as tetrahydrocannabinol (THC), found in marijuana. Ambitious research is necessary to understand fully how these substances affect the human body.
- Experts who have dealt with all available data do not recommend that the goal of research should be smoked marijuana for medical conditions. Rather, they support development of a smoke-free, rapid-onset delivery system for compounds found in the plant.

In 1997, the National Institutes of Health (NIH) met "to review the scientific data concerning the potential therapeutic uses of marijuana and the need for and feasibility of additional research." The collection of experts had experience in relevant studies and clinical research, but held no preconceived opinions about the medical use of marijuana. They were asked the following questions: What is the current state of scientific knowledge; what significant questions remain unanswered; what is the medical potential; what possible uses deserve further research; and what issues should be considered if clinical trials are conducted?

Shortly thereafter, the White House Office of National Drug Control Policy (ONDCP) asked the Institute of Medicine (IOM) to execute a similar task: To form a panel that would "conduct a review of the scientific evidence to assess the potential health benefits and risks of marijuana and its constituent cannabinoids." Selected reviewers were among the most accomplished in the disciplines of neuroscience, pharmacology, immunology, drug abuse, drug laws, oncology, infectious diseases, and ophthalmology. Their analysis focused on the effects of isolated cannabinoids, risks associated with medical use of marijuana, and the use of smoked marijuana. Their findings in the IOM study stated:

Compared to most drugs, the accumulation of medical knowledge about marijuana has proceeded in reverse. Typically,
during the course of drug development, a compound is first
found to have some medical benefit. Following this, extensive
tests are undertaken to determine the safety and proper dose
of the drug for medical use. Marijuana, in contrast, has been
widely used in the United States for decades. . . . The data on
the adverse effects of marijuana are more extensive than the
data on effectiveness. Clinical studies of marijuana are difficult to conduct.

Nevertheless, the IOM report concluded that cannabinoid drugs
do have potential for therapeutic use. It specifically named pain,
nausea and vomiting, and lack of appetite as symptoms for which
cannabinoids may be of benefit, stating that cannabinoids are
"moderately well suited" for AIDS wasting and nausea resulting
from chemotherapy. The report found that cannabinoids "probably
have a natural role in pain modulation, control of movement, and
memory," but that this role "is likely to be multi-faceted and
remains unclear."

Evaluating the Medical Uses of Marijuana

In addressing the possible effects of smoked marijuana on pain, the
NIH report explained that no clinical trials involving patients with
"naturally occurring pain" have ever been conducted but that two
credible studies of cancer pain indicated analgesic benefit. Addressing another possible benefit—the reduction of nausea related to
chemotherapy—the NIH report described a study comparing oral
administration of THC (via a drug called Dronabinol) and smoked
marijuana. Of 20 patients, nine expressed no preference between the
two, seven preferred the oral THC, and only four preferred smoked
marijuana. In summary, the report states, "No scientific questions
have been definitively answered about the efficacy of smoked marijuana in chemotherapy-related nausea and vomiting."

In the area of glaucoma, the effect of marijuana on intraocular
pressure (the cause of optic nerve damage that typifies glaucoma) was
explored, and smoked marijuana was found to reduce this pressure.
However, the NIH report failed to find evidence that marijuana can
"safely and effectively lower intraocular pressure enough to prevent
optic nerve damage." The report concluded that the "mechanism of
action" of smoked marijuana or THC in pill form on intraocular pressure is not known and calls for more research.

In addressing appetite stimulation and wasting related to AIDS,
the NIH report recognized the potential benefit of marijuana. However, the report also noted the lack of pertinent data. The researchers
pointed out that the evidence known to date, although plentiful, is
anecdotal, and "no objective data relative to body composition alter-

ations, HIV replication, or immunologic function in HIV patients are available."

Smoking marijuana as medicine was recommended by neither report. The IOM report called smoked marijuana a "crude THC delivery system" that is not recommended because it delivers harmful substances, pointing out that botanical products are susceptible to problems with consistency, contaminations, uncertain potencies, and instabilities. The NIH report reached the same conclusion and explained that eliminating the smoked aspect of marijuana would "remove an important obstacle" from research into the potential medical benefits of the plant.

These studies present a consistent theme: Cannabinoids in marijuana do show potential for symptom management of several conditions, but research is inadequate to explain definitively how cannabinoids operate to deliver these potential benefits. Nor did the studies attribute any curative effects to marijuana; at best, only the symptoms of particular medical conditions are affected. The finding most important to the debate is that the studies did not advocate smoked marijuana as medicine. To the contrary, the NIH report called for a non-smoked alternative as a focus of further research. The IOM report recommended smoking marijuana as medicine only in the most extreme circumstances when all other medication has failed and then only when administration of marijuana is under strict medical supervision.

These conclusions from two studies, based not on rhetorical conjecture but on credible scientific research, do not support the legalization of smoked marijuana as medicine.

The Scientific Community's Views

The conclusions of the NIH and IOM reports are supported by commentary published in the nation's medical journals. Much of this literature focuses on the problematic aspect of smoke as a delivery system when using cannabinoids for medical purposes. One physician-authored article describes smoking "crude plant material" as "troublesome" to many doctors and "unpleasant" to many patients. Dr. Eric Voth, chairman of the International Drug Strategy Institute, stated in a 1997 article published in the *Journal of the American Medical Association* (*JAMA*): "To support research on smoked pot does not make sense. We're currently in a huge anti-tobacco thrust in this country, which is appropriate. So why should we waste money on drug delivery that is based on smoking?" Voth recommends non-smoked analogs to THC.

In September 1998, the editor in chief of the *New England Journal of Medicine*, Dr. Jerome P. Kassirer, in a coauthored piece with Dr. Marcia Angell, wrote:

Until the 20th century, most remedies were botanical, a few

of which were found through trial and error to be helpful. All of that began to change in the 20th century as a result of rapid advances in medical science. In particular, the evolution of the randomized, controlled clinical trial enabled researchers to study with precision the safety, efficacy, and dose effects of proposed treatments and the indications for them. No longer do we have to rely on trial and error and anecdotes. We have learned to ask and expect statistically reliable evidence before accepting conclusions about remedies.

Dr. Robert DuPont of the Georgetown University Department of Psychiatry points out that those who aggressively advocate smoking marijuana as medicine "undermine" the potentially beneficial roles of the NIH and IOM studies. As does Dr. Voth, DuPont discusses the possibility of non-smoked delivery methods. He asserts that if the scientific community were to accept smoked marijuana as medicine, the public would likely perceive the decision as influenced by politics rather than science. DuPont concludes that if research is primarily concerned with the needs of the sick, it is unlikely that science will approve of smoked marijuana as medicine.

Even those who advocate smoking marijuana for medicine are occasionally driven to caution. Dr. Lester Grinspoon, a Harvard University professor and advocate of smoking marijuana, warned in a 1994 *JAMA* article: "The one area we have to be concerned about is pulmonary function. The lungs were not made to inhale anything but fresh air." Other experts have only disdain for the loose medical claims for smoked marijuana. Dr. Janet Lapey, executive director of Concerned Citizens for Drug Prevention, likened research on smoked marijuana to using opium pipes to test morphine. She advocates research on isolated active compounds rather than smoked marijuana.

The findings of the NIH and IOM reports, and other commentary by members of the scientific and medical communities, contradict the idea that plant smoking is an appropriate vehicle for delivering whatever compounds research may find to be of benefit.

The FDA Evaluation

The mission of the Food and Drug Administration's (FDA) Center for Drug Evaluation and Research is "to assure that safe and effective drugs are available to the American people." Circumvention of the FDA approval process would remove this essential safety mechanism intended to safeguard public health. The FDA approval process is not designed to keep drugs out of the hands of the sick but to offer a system to ensure that drugs prevent, cure, or treat a medical condition. FDA approval can involve testing of hundreds of compounds, which allows scientists to alter them for improved performance. The IOM report addresses this situation explicitly: "Medicines today are expected to be of known composition and quantity. Even in cases where marijuana can provide relief from symptoms, the crude plant mixture does not meet this modern expectation."

For a proposed drug to gain approval by the FDA, a potential manufacturer must produce a new drug application. The application must provide enough information for FDA reviewers to determine (among other criteria) "whether the drug is safe and effective for its proposed use(s), whether the benefits of the drug outweigh its risks [and] whether the methods used in manufacturing the drug and the controls used to maintain the drug's quality are adequate to preserve the drug's integrity, strength, quality, and purity."

On the "benefits" side, the Institute of Medicine found that the therapeutic effects of cannabinoids are "generally modest" and that for the majority of symptoms there are approved drugs that are more effective. For example, superior glaucoma and anti-nausea medications have already been developed. In addition, the new drug Zofran may provide more relief than THC for chemotherapy patients. Dronabinol, the synthetic THC, offers immunocompromised HIV patients a safe alternative to inhaling marijuana smoke, which contains carcinogens.

On the "risks" side, there is strong evidence that smoking marijuana has detrimental health effects. Unrefined marijuana contains approximately 400 chemicals that become combustible when smoked, producing in turn over 2,000 impure chemicals. These substances, many of which remain unidentified, include carcinogens. The IOM report states that, when used chronically, "marijuana smoking is associated with abnormalities of cells lining the human respiratory tract. Marijuana smoke, like tobacco smoke, is associated with increased risk of cancer, lung damage, and poor pregnancy outcomes." A subsequent study by Dr. Zuo-Feng Zhary of the Jonsson Cancer Center at the University of California at Los Angeles (UCLA) determined that the carcinogens in marijuana are much stronger than those in tobacco.

Chronic bronchitis and increased incidence of pulmonary disease are associated with frequent use of smoked marijuana, as are reduced sperm motility and testosterone levels in males. Decreased immune system response, which is likely to increase vulnerability to infection and tumors, is also associated with frequent use. Even a slight decrease in immune response can have major public health ramifications. Because marijuana by-products remain in body fat for several weeks, interference with normal body functioning may continue beyond the time of use. Among the known effects of smoking marijuana is impaired lung function similar to the type caused by cigarette smoking.

In addressing the efficacy of cannabinoid drugs, the IOM report— after recognizing "potential therapeutic value"—added that smoked marijuana is "a crude THC delivery system that also delivers harmful substances." Purified cannabinoid compounds are preferable to plants in crude form, which contain inconsistent chemical composition. The "therapeutic window" between the desirable and adverse effects of marijuana and THC is narrow at best and may not exist at all, in many cases.

The scientific evidence that marijuana's potential therapeutic benefits are modest, that other approved drugs are generally more effective, and that smoking marijuana is unhealthy, indicates that smoked marijuana is not a viable candidate for FDA approval. Without such approval, smoked marijuana cannot achieve legitimate status as an approved drug that patients can readily use. This reality renders the advocacy of smoking marijuana as medicine both misguided and impractical.

Mixing Politics and Medicine

While ballot initiatives are an indispensable part of our democracy, they are imprudent in the context of advancing smoked marijuana as medicine because they confound our system of laws, create conflict between state and federal law, and fail to offer a proper substitute for science.

Ballot initiatives to legalize smoking marijuana as medicine have had a tumultuous history. In 1998 alone, initiatives were passed in five states, but any substantive benefits in the aftermath were lacking. For example, a Colorado proposal was ruled invalid before the election. An Ohio bill was passed but subsequently repealed. In the District of Colombia, Congress disallowed the counting of ballot results. Six other states permit patients to smoke marijuana as medicine but only by prescription, and doctors, dubious about the validity of a smoked medicine, wary of liability suits, and concerned about legal and professional risks are reluctant to prescribe it for their patients. Although voters passed Arizona's initiative, the state legislature originally blocked the measure. The version that eventually became Arizona law is problematic because it conflicts with federal statute.

Indeed, legalization at the state level creates a direct conflict between state and federal law in every case, placing patients, doctors, police, prosecutors, and public officials in a difficult position. The fundamental legal problem with prescription of marijuana is that federal law prohibits such use, rendering state law functionally ineffective.

To appreciate fully the legal ramifications of ballot initiatives, consider one specific example. California's is perhaps the most publicized, and illustrates the chaos that can result from such initiatives. Enacted in 1996, the California Compassionate Use Act (also known as Proposition 215) was a ballot initiative intended to afford legal protection to seriously ill patients who use marijuana therapeutically. The act explicitly states that marijuana used by patients must first be recommended by a physician, and refers to such use as a "right" of the people of California. According to the act, physicians and patients are not subject to prosecution if they are compliant with the terms of the legislation. The act names cancer, anorexia, aids, chronic pain, spasticity, glaucoma, arthritis, and migraine as conditions that may be appropriately treated by marijuana, but it also includes the proviso: "or any other illness for which marijuana provides relief."

Writing in December 1999, a California doctor, Ryan Thompson, summed up the medical problems with Proposition 215:

As it stands, it creates vague, ill-defined guidelines that are obviously subject to abuse. The most glaring areas are as follows:

- A patient does not necessarily need to be seen, evaluated or diagnosed as having any specific medical condition to qualify for the use of marijuana.
- There is no requirement for a written prescription or even a written recommendation for its medical use.
- Once "recommended," the patient never needs to be seen again to assess the effectiveness of the treatment and potentially could use that "recommendation" for the rest of his or her life.
- There is no limitation to the conditions for which it can be used, it can be recommended for virtually any condition, even if it is not believed to be effective.

The doctor concludes by stating: "Certainly as a physician I have witnessed the detrimental effects of marijuana use on patients and their families. It is not a harmless substance."

A Conflict Between State and Federal Law

Passage of Proposition 215 resulted in conflict between California and the federal government. In February 1997, the Executive Office of the President issued its response to the California Compassionate Use Act (as well as Arizona's Proposition 200). The notice stated:

[The] Department of Justice's (DOJ) position is that a practitioner's practice of recommending or prescribing Schedule I controlled substances is not consistent with the public interest (as that phrase is used in the federal Controlled Substances Act) and will lead to administrative action by the Drug Enforcement Administration (DEA) to revoke the practitioner's registration.

The notice indicated that U.S. attorneys in California and Arizona would consider cases for prosecution using certain criteria. These included lack of a bona fide doctor-patient relationship, a "high volume" of prescriptions (or recommendations) for Schedule I drugs, "significant" profits derived from such prescriptions, prescriptions to minors, and "special circumstances" like impaired driving accidents involving serious injury.

The federal government's reasons for taking such a stance are solid. Dr. Donald Vereen of the Office of National Drug Control Policy explains that "research-based evidence" must be the focus when evaluating the risks and benefits of any drug, the only approach that provides a rational basis for making such a determination. He also explains that since testing by the Food and Drug Administration and other government agencies are designed to protect public health, circumvention of the process is unwise.

While the federal government supports FDA approved cannabinoid-based drugs, it maintains that ballot initiatives should not be allowed to remove marijuana evaluation from the realm of science and the drug approval process—a position based on a concern for public health. The Department of Health and Human Services has revised its regulations by making research-grade marijuana more available and intends to facilitate more research of cannabinoids. The department does not, however, intend to lower its standards of scientific proof.

Problems resulting from the California initiative are not isolated to conflict between the state and federal government. California courts themselves limited the distribution of medical marijuana. A 1997 California Appellate decision held that the state's Compassionate Use Act only allowed purchase of medical marijuana from a patient's "primary caregiver," not from "drug dealers on street corners" or "sales centers such as the Cannabis Buyers' Club." This decision allowed courts to enjoin marijuana clubs.

The course of California's initiative and those of other states illustrate that such ballot-driven movements are not a legally effective or reliable way to supply the sick with whatever medical benefit the marijuana plant might hold. If the focus were shifted away from smoking the plant and toward a non-smoked alternative based on scientific research, much of this conflict could be avoided.

Filling "Prescriptions"

It is one thing to pass a ballot initiative defining a burning plant as medicine. It is yet another to make available such "medicine" if the plant itself remains—as it should—illegal. Recreational use, after all, cannot be equated with medicinal use, and none of the ballots passed were constructed to do so.

Nonetheless, cannabis buyers' clubs were quick to present the fiction that, for medical benefit, they were now in business to provide relief for the sick. In California, 13 such clubs rapidly went into operation, selling marijuana openly under the guise that doing so had been legitimized at the polls. The problem was that these organizations were selling to people under the flimsiest of facades. One club went so far as to proclaim: "All use of marijuana is medical. It makes you smarter. It touches the right brain and allows you to slow down, to smell the flowers."

Depending on the wording of the specific ballots, legal interpretation of what was allowed became problematic. The buyers' clubs became notorious for liberal interpretations of "prescription," "doctor's recommendation," and "medical." In California, Lucy Mae Tuck obtained a prescription for marijuana to treat hot flashes. Another citizen arrested for possession claimed he was medically entitled to his stash to treat a condition exacerbated by an ingrown toenail. Undercover police in several buyers' clubs reported blatant sales to minors and adults with little attention to claims of medical need or a doctor's direction. Eventually, 10 of the 13 clubs in California were closed.

Further exacerbating the confusion over smoked marijuana as medicine are doctors' concerns over medical liability. Without the Food and Drug Administration's approval, marijuana cannot become a pharmaceutical drug to be purchased at local drug stores. Nor can there be any degree of confidence that proper doses can be measured out and chemical impurities eliminated in the marijuana that is obtained. After all, we are talking about a leaf, and a burning one at that. In the meantime, the harmful effects of marijuana have been documented in greater scientific detail than any findings about the medical benefits of smoking the plant.

Given the serious illnesses (for example, cancer and AIDS) of some of those who are purported to be in need of smoked marijuana for medical relief and their vulnerability to impurities and other toxic substances present in the plant, doctors are loath to risk their patients' health and their own financial well-being by prescribing it. As Dr. Peter Byeff, an oncologist at a Connecticut cancer center, points out: "If there's no mechanism for dispensing it, that doesn't help many of my patients. They're not going to go out and grow it in their backyards." Recognizing the availability of effective prescription medications to control nausea and vomiting, Byeff adds: "There's no reason to prescribe or dispense marijuana."

Medical professionals recognize what marijuana-as-medicine advocates seek to obscure. The chemical makeup of any two marijuana plants can differ significantly due to minor variations in cultivation. For example, should one plant receive relative to another as little as four more hours of collective sunlight before cultivation, the two could turn out to be significantly different in chemical composition. Potency also varies according to climate and geographical origin; it can also be affected by the way in which the plant is harvested and stored. Differences can be so profound that under current medical standards, two marijuana plants could be considered completely different drugs. Prescribing unproven, unmeasured, impure burnt leaves to relieve symptoms of a wide range of ailments does not seem to be the high point of American medical practice.

A Counterproductive Measure

Cannabinoids found in the marijuana plant offer the potential for medical use. However, lighting the leaves of the plant on fire and smoking them amount to an impractical delivery system that involves health risks and deleterious legal consequences. There is a profound difference between an approval process that seeks to purify isolated compounds for safe and effective delivery, and legalization of smoking the raw plant material as medicine. To advocate the latter is to bypass the safety and efficacy built into America's medical system. Ballot initiatives for smoked marijuana comprise a dangerous, impractical shortcut that circumvents the drug-approval process. The resulting decriminalization of a dangerous and harmful drug turns out to be counterproductive—legally, politically, and scientifically.

Advocacy for smoked marijuana has been cast in terms of relief from suffering. The Hippocratic oath that doctors take specifies that they must "first, do no harm." Clearly some people supporting medical marijuana are genuinely concerned about the sick. But violating established medical procedure does do harm, and it confounds the political, medical, and legal processes that best serve American society. In the single-minded pursuit of an extreme position that harkens back to an era of home medicine and herbal remedies, advocates for smoked marijuana as medicinal therapy not only retard legitimate scientific progress but become easy prey for less noble-minded zealots who seek to promote the acceptance and use of marijuana, an essentially harmful—and, therefore, illegal—drug.

CHAPTER 4

PERSONAL STORIES OF THE USE AND ABUSE OF MARIJUANA

Contemporary Issues
Companion

Marijuana Addiction: One Family's Nightmare

Ronald G. Shafer

> On October 1, 1987, sixteen-year-old Ryan Shafer was killed in an automobile accident while high on drugs. Ryan's father, Ronald G. Shafer, describes the harrowing facts of his son's drug addiction in the following selection. Shafer explains that his son first began using marijuana and then turned to harder drugs. When Shafer and his wife discovered Ryan's addiction, they placed him in a drug treatment program. Ryan seemed to be recovering at first, Shafer writes, but then he started to use marijuana and other drugs again. According to Shafer, parents often minimize the seriousness of their children's marijuana use because they believe it is not a dangerous drug. However, he maintains, many experts consider marijuana a gateway to the abuse of more dangerous drugs such as LSD—the drug which ultimately led to his own son's death. Shafer is a staff reporter for the *Wall Street Journal*.

America's new nightmare is our children as victims of drugs.

My teenage son, Ryan, started using drugs at about age 12. He played Little League baseball, had a sunny smile and big brown eyes, and was a free-spirited person who could make you laugh. He collected baseball cards. Now, Ryan's laughter is gone. Because of drugs, he is dead. And every day, my heart breaks a little more.

My family and I are reliving our nightmare in the hope that it might save another young person who thinks he or she can control their drug use. We may help a family from experiencing the pain we will always feel.

Discovering the Problem

As a parent I am amazed that our children can hide even extreme drug and alcohol abuse from us until it is almost too late. We did not find out about Ryan's drug use until he was 14. And the extent of his use was far beyond our worst fears. I recently learned from Ryan's notes about his drug use in 1986: "I used cocaine a lot. It started out as a weekend use, but soon I had or tried to have it daily. I used PCP (a

Reprinted from "America's Nightmare—Youth and Drugs: A Personal Experience," opening address of the National Conference on Marijuana Use: Prevention, Treatment and Research, delivered by Ronald G. Shafer on July 19, 1995.

hallucinogen) two or three times a week. I used hallucinogens all the time, such as acid, mushrooms, peyote, ecstasy, and mescaline. I used LSD about 300 times." It was marijuana that started Ryan on his downfall and was always the drug he went back to.

Most people never intend to get addicted to drugs. I am sure that Ryan never meant to get hooked. Ryan Glenn Shafer came into our lives on May 27, 1971, when my wife Barbara and I adopted him. He was 2 months old, and a major expansion to our family.

Ryan became a boy with wide and intense interests, who was fun-loving, had a sense of humor, and charmed his friends and adults. Ryan had been troubled by low self-esteem and by difficulty in school, despite being named "Joe Cool" at his school. (We now know that both are early warning signs of a child at risk of drug use.) We now know that Ryan had begun experimenting with drugs as early as the sixth grade. While Ryan went through his stages of drug abuse, we were going through the typical stages of parents of drug-abusing adolescents.

The Stages Parents Go Through

The first stage is ignorance. In 1983 we never suspected that drug use was possible with our preteen. He was way too young. We began to notice personality changes, hostility, and rebellion. These seemed to be normal changes we had seen in our friends' teenagers.

The next stage is denial. Ryan's actions worsened, but we did not accept what we know now were warning signs: use of eye drops to cover up red eyes from smoking marijuana, incense burning in his room to mask the odor, calls from friends whom we had not met, trouble at school, money missing from around the house.

In 1985 Ryan, in the ninth grade, could no longer hide his drug troubles. He began cutting classes—a common tipoff to drug use. He had missed nearly two dozen classes and was failing everything by the time the school called us. School officials at that time did not know much more about drugs than we did.

The school did guide us to a local physician who had treated hundreds of adolescents. Ryan denied drug use as most drug abusers do. "You don't trust me," he self-righteously protested.

Tests showed "low positive" for marijuana use. His tests would have been "high positive," but Ryan was sneaking into our bedroom and watering his urine. He later informed us of this and that he had been cutting classes to smoke marijuana daily.

The next stage was minimization. Thank God, it was "only" pot. Marijuana can be a damaging drug for young people. Heavy use can cause short-term memory loss and long-term health problems. Pot and alcohol can also be gateways to more serious drugs. By now, Ryan was long past his experimental stage of drug use and was into planned use.

As Ryan advanced into his third stage of drug abuse, chemical dependence, his problems took control of our family. Drugs changed him into a person we did not recognize. He was lying, shouting, scheming, and manipulating. My wife and I experienced anger over his actions, uncertainty over his insistence that he was innocent, and frustration over our inability to resolve the situation. It was time for professional help.

Seeking Professional Help

In January 1986, we moved into the stage of acceptance and placed Ryan in the Arlington (VA) Hospital's 6-week, residential, adolescent treatment program. When Ryan hit bottom he was ready to accept treatment. Despite this, he still hid the full extent of his use from us. He told us later that he saw snakes coming out of the TV set the night before entering treatment, while [appearing] to be calm. He was on an LSD "acid trip." The intake tests revealed the extent of his drug use. He was called a "garbage head," a person who heavily abuses both drugs and alcohol.

Ryan's drug of choice was LSD, which causes vivid hallucinations. Fellow residents called him "blotter boy" because he had used LSD impregnated on blotter paper and sold like sheets of stamps for as little as $3 to $5 a hit.

We discovered the limits of drug testing. LSD is detectable only in special tests, while cocaine remains in the system for about 2 to 3 days. Marijuana stays in the system about 30 days and thus is the most likely to be detected.

While Ryan received treatment, Barb and I attended parent-counseling sessions. We learned that, like us, most parents had no idea of their children's heavy drug or alcohol use until the youths could no longer hide their dual lives. Some of the parents were strict, some were lenient, all were caring. Most were middle-class with insurance. There is no magic bullet of parenting against drugs.

Ryan dove into the program with gusto. He won over counselors and parents with his charm. We finally got our real son back. He told us about how he had slipped out of his bedroom window at night to buy drugs. Ryan was home for his 15th birthday in March 1986. He attended 15 weeks of after-care 5 days a week. He went to the 90 meetings of Alcoholics Anonymous or Narcotics Anonymous as required. He was on the road to recovery and our troubles were behind us.

Ryan was a 10th-grader by his 16th birthday, and was doing great. His drug tests were clean and his grades were great. He raised his reading level, damaged by pot use, to 12th-grade level; got his driver's license, and worked part-time. It was a joy having our son back.

Suddenly, the old signs reappeared. His grades dropped, he spent money excessively, and his behavior deteriorated. A test showed signs of marijuana, probably laced with PCP. Ryan had to go into another rehab program. We were crushed.

In spring 1987, he entered a new 10-week outpatient program at Arlington Hospital. As he progressed, his tests showed no drugs, but his personality did not return. He remained abusive and temper prone.

We believe he truly wanted to stop using drugs. In a note he wrote, thanking us for putting him in treatment, he said: "For the first time in a long time I am very happy with my life. I really do not want to lose what I have just because I want to smoke pot."

Then the situation took a dark turn. Ryan became involved with a person he claimed to be his Alcoholics Anonymous "sponsor." He was supposed to be a recovering addict with more sober time who could help Ryan. We discovered the man to be connected with Ryan's earlier drug use. We forbade Ryan from seeing the man, but he did so anyway. Things began to deteriorate quickly.

Ryan talked about committing suicide for the first time. He was ejected from the rehab program the next day after testing positive for marijuana. Springwood Psychiatric Hospital had one bed open. We took him in that night.

This time Ryan resisted. We got him to Springwood, where doctors told us he was in a deep depression. Therapy indicated low self-esteem. He was diagnosed a manic-depressive, suffering the wide mood swings of a bipolar disorder. It is not known whether drugs caused his problems, or whether he used drugs to self-medicate. Tests at Springwood showed no recent drug use and there were no withdrawal symptoms, but with LSD there are not any.

Once again, he responded to treatment. His mood swings were stabilized with lithium and other medicines. After 6 weeks, in early September, he came home. He was accepted at Fairfax County's special education school.

Ryan seemed free from drugs and more like his old self. He closely followed the news and discussed the Supreme Court nomination of Robert Bork. He would correct his father, the journalist, with, "I think I know a little bit more about Supreme Court nominations than you do."

His medicine made him tired, and he often went to bed early. One night in late September, I looked in his room and said, "I love you, Ryan." He picked his head up, smiled, and said softly, "Thanks, Dad."

The Death of a Son

Within the week, he was dead. The fatal accident occurred at about 8:30 p.m. on October 1, 1987. It hit us with a jolt of electricity: Ryan was dead. I would never hold my little boy again. It is true that if your child dies, a part of you dies with him.

Ryan drove his car off a street in Vienna, VA. He inexplicably fled the minor accident and ran a half-mile down the road, where he was bumped by a car. This motorist tried to help Ryan, but he resisted and continued inexplicably fleeing. Ryan ran onto another highway where he was hit head-on and killed instantly by a van. This vehicle did not even stop.

Tests showed no evidence of drugs. But Ryan, we learned, was speeding from the home of a drug dealer. Ryan had obtained LSD, a hallucinogen that can cause panic and that often does not show up in tests, from someone earlier in the day. One way or another, drugs took my only son.

In the suburbs of America, both drug use and the violence related to it are often hidden. Ryan was coming from the home of a drug dealer. Several young people came forward to police after Ryan's death. These accounts along with our pleas resulted in the drug dealer's arrest. He was charged with distributing marijuana and other drugs to minors. He also was charged with the statutory rape of a 13-year-old girl and with soliciting sex from a 14-year-old boy.

Our main concern after Ryan's death was the psychological impact on our daughter, Katie, now nearly 16. Katie has never used drugs and has dealt with the loss of her brother by counseling others against drug use.

The key to saving lives is early intervention, during the first to third years that young people typically hide their drug use. If you feel in your heart something is not right, it is better to get your child in for an evaluation.

The only real solution is prevention. We must keep kids from ever trying drugs in the first place. Drug education—as early as elementary school—is vital, and it should include parents and teachers.

Countless deaths of youth like Ryan are related to drugs and are not recorded in the Nation's rising drug toll.

I will never fully know why Ryan got involved in drugs. In my view, there is still a dangerous myth that good kids from good families do not do drugs. Children are vulnerable no matter who they are or where they live. My son had his problems, but he was a sensitive, caring, and unforgettable young man. Now we visit Ryan's grave and we weep, and we ask, Why?

For Ryan, it is too late. It may not be too late for your children.

I Broke the Law to Save My Son

Cheryl Johnson, as told to Steve Rubenstein

In the following selection, Cheryl Johnson relates her family's experience with the medical use of marijuana. Johnson's teenage son, Simon, has Crohn's disease, which causes nausea and vomiting. Only marijuana has proven effective at alleviating his symptoms, Johnson asserts. Johnson admits that she and her husband were angry when they first discovered Simon was smoking marijuana, but when they saw how well marijuana controlled the debilitative symptoms of his illness, they began to view marijuana as medicine, not as an illegal drug. Although they live in California, which has legalized the medical use of marijuana, Johnson explains that most doctors are still reluctant to prescribe marijuana due to federal laws criminalizing it, so they are forced to obtain Simon's marijuana illegally. Johnson fears arrest, but she sees no other alternative except to continue providing her son the marijuana that allows him to lead a normal life. Steve Rubenstein is a staff writer for the *San Francisco Chronicle*. The family's names have been changed to protect their privacy.

We're the most normal family you could imagine. We mail in our taxes on time, and we always stop at red lights. We never take more than ten items through the express checkout lane. We've got a basketball hoop out front and a swimming pool in back. I'm a troop leader for the Girl Scouts. And every morning, I send my 17-year-old son to school with marijuana in his backpack.

Never in a million years would I have chosen to do this. But in my heart I know that marijuana is helping Simon get on with his life. You see, he has Crohn's Disease, an incurable and painful inflammation of the intestinal tract that can cause life-threatening complications. Simon is plagued with nausea and vomiting, and the only thing that relieves them is marijuana.

So, Simon uses marijuana with our blessing. I even bought him a lipstick holder in which to keep his daily supply—though he has to be careful no one sees him using it. A law was passed here in California permitting the use of marijuana for medicinal purposes, but federal law still forbids its sale or use under any circumstances.

I think it's important for people to know that my husband, Dave, and I aren't weird, or overly permissive parents. In addition to Simon, our middle child, we have two daughters—Marie, 19, and Julie, 11. We live in a middle-class neighborhood in San Jose. Dave is a manager for a computer company, where he's worked for 16 years and I've been a radiology supervisor at a hospital for 21 years.

An Illness Develops

The first time Simon got sick, he was 6 years old. His first-grade teacher told us he was trying to avoid doing homework by faking stomachaches. But then he started throwing up so often that his doctor had him admitted to the hospital. After three weeks of tests, the results were inconclusive.

Simon spontaneously recovered, and went on just fine. He was an outgoing kid—quick with clever one-liners, someone who cheered you up just by being around him. His medical ordeal seemed over, and we gratefully put it behind us.

It wasn't until he was 13 that he began complaining of severe stomachaches again. Over a couple of months, I'd begun to notice that he was getting really pale and lethargic. Then he started throwing up, and I took him to the doctor, determined to get a definite diagnosis.

Simon's condition worsened, and he was hospitalized—this time for a month. Finally, we were told he had Crohn's Disease. We'll never know if he had the illness when he was 6 and his doctors simply missed it or if he had ulcers, which was their best guess at the time. In any case, we now knew for sure that he had a devastating disease, and we were very worried. The doctors said they didn't know if the disease was hereditary; as far as we can trace, there's no history of it in our family. Simon was put on Prednisone, a powerful steroid that controls the inflammation but can be taken for only a limited time.

He would improve while on the drug, then get sick when he had to stop taking it. When Simon was 15, he developed other symptoms—a high fever, pancreatitis, anemia, internal bleeding—any of which could have been fatal. For two months, he lay in a hospital bed being fed intravenously. Dave, Marie, and Julie would come to see him every afternoon. I rarely left the hospital. All I could think about was how unfair it was that my sweet, funny boy was going to have to deal with this cruel disease for the rest of his life.

Finally, the doctors put him on a drug that seemed to control the disease—the immune-suppressant 6-Mercaptopurine. Unfortunately, it exacerbated the nausea and vomiting. Simon tried a number of prescription antinausea remedies, but they either didn't help or made him groggy. After his release from the hospital, he had to stay home from school for a month, and was so sick and depressed he didn't want to be around anyone. Who could blame him?

A Source of Relief from Pain and Nausea

On his own, Simon found a way out of his misery. While still in the hospital, he'd heard that some cancer patients smoke marijuana to relieve their pain. It's not hard for a high school kid to get marijuana— it's everywhere. He bought some from a schoolmate, and tried it.

We began to notice that he seemed to feel better at times, yet we didn't understand why. But Simon didn't want to answer our questions; in fact, he started to withdraw from us more and more. He became secretive, someone we hardly recognized—sneaking out of the house at odd hours, barely talking to us at all. He was also hanging out with kids we suspected were drug users, and his grades dropped drastically.

Dave and I found out what was going on in the worst possible way: A school counselor found Simon sneaking a puff behind the tennis court and called the police, who came and arrested him. He was immediately expelled and reassigned to another school in the district.

The moment I found out about the marijuana, I went ballistic. I screamed and yelled and lectured Simon, without giving him a chance to explain. All I knew was that we'd always taught our children that it's stupid to use drugs, and here, I thought, was my son getting stoned!

My reaction scared him so much that he couldn't tell us the truth: that he *needed* the marijuana and feared we'd take it away and start watching his every move. In a calmer mood, Dave sat down with him and told him he had to give it up. At that, Simon cried and said he couldn't—and why.

We changed our minds once we saw that the marijuana really helped to control his nausea and vomiting. And Simon didn't have to get high—he could keep the dosage at a relatively low level.

Support from the Family

Simon's troubles were hardly over. He was afraid to take the marijuana to his new school, where he often felt so sick he'd have to put his head down on his desk. He tried to explain why he couldn't raise his head, but the teacher thought he was just being disrespectful. And because he'd entered the school on probation, it took only these minor incidents for him to be expelled again. I was furious, and decided we had to make school officials understand what Simon was up against. Together, Dave, Simon, and I called on the principal at Simon's first school and explained his illness. He was accepted back. Soon his grades improved, he got a part-time job, his friends changed. He was our Simon again, the boy we've always loved.

We limited how much marijuana Simon had at any given time

because we didn't want him to get into trouble or give any to his friends. He started keeping a small amount in a plastic Baggie in his room, and that's the only place in the house that he's allowed to use it. He takes a few puffs in the morning, another dose midday—always off school premises—and a final one at night. I keep a larger bag in my room. He knows where it is, and he's proven to us that this is something we can trust him with.

Now that our family is pulling together, we've become a tighter, tougher unit. We've made every Tuesday evening family night, no matter what. We either go out to dinner or a movie or just sit around playing a game. We know we can count on each other when it matters.

Dave and I have explained to our daughters what Simon is doing and why, and they've been very supportive. Simon's older sister, Marie, used to drive him to school every morning and would have to stop on the way so he could throw up. When he was in the hospital a couple of years ago, she answered questions about his health from teachers and kids—which was tough because she was scared he was going to die. Now, she's become his champion; in her last year of high school she wrote a paper explaining why she believes that marijuana should be legalized for medicinal purposes.

Obtaining a Controversial Medicine

Because we hated the idea of Simon having to buy marijuana on his own, we started taking him to the Cannabis Cultivators Club in San Francisco. It's a 90-minute drive each way from our home, so it takes the whole day just to get his medicine—the kind of errand most people can do by just popping into the corner drugstore. We take the girls along on these monthly trips and make a day of it by going shopping in the city or taking in the sights. The club requires a doctor's letter, which we got from Simon's gastroenterologist.

We got scared early in 1996, when state drug-enforcement officers raided the club and shut it down. For awhile, we thought we'd be forced to buy Simon's marijuana on the street, risking arrest and God knows what else. When I told my friends and coworkers about his problem, a number of them came up and whispered that they could get marijuana for me. It seemed as if everyone knew how to put their hands on it but me!

But in November 1996, after California residents approved Proposition 215 allowing the medicinal use of marijuana, the cultivators club reopened. Still, we're in a catch-22: Though a doctor in California can now "recommend" marijuana as a health-care regimen for a specific illness, the American Medical Association warns that a doctor who does so risks having his license to prescribe *any* drug revoked by the Justice Department's Drug Enforcement Agency.

I have to say, when I look at Simon's plastic bag, I don't see something legal or illegal. I see medicine—medicine my son needs to live a full life. And that's what he's trying to do, under tough circumstances.

Simon has a special gift for understanding other people's pain. Recently, he heard about the wife of a friend of mine who was suffering from nausea brought on by chemotherapy. Her doctor had recommended marijuana, but she didn't know where to get it. Simon knew what this woman was going through, so he divided his supply and gave half to her. I was proud of him.

The idea of any of us being arrested by federal drug agents and going to jail is terrifying. But if there are options out there that we haven't tried, I'd like to know what they are.

These days, we're just happy that Simon is busy with the same things as other boys his age. He's starting his senior year in high school now. He likes to dunk basketballs on the court out front. Even though Simon has tried to explain the situation to his friends, they don't always get it. Sometimes they tease him and say, "You're so lucky. Your mom lets you smoke pot." He has mood swings like most teenagers—days when he seems to need his family and days when he doesn't want anything to do with us. He doesn't like his parents telling him what to wear or hanging around when his friends are over—which sounds like your typical 17-year-old. He loves computers and plans to attend a computer training school after he graduates. Hopefully, he will have a normal life span—most Crohn's patients do.

Simon still has serious medical problems. The 6-Mercaptopurine can cause liver damage, so he has to have his blood tested monthly. The current plan is to keep him on the drug for as long as it continues to be effective and doesn't harm him. We're keeping our fingers crossed. We do a lot of that in our house.

I've never thought of myself as a crusader. But I know I'm not crazy, and I'm not a criminal either. I'm just a mom who's doing the best she can for her family. Because that's what moms do.

AN ACTIVIST FOR MEDICAL MARIJUANA

Linda Peterson

In November 1996, Californians approved Proposition 215, the medical marijuana initiative that exempts from prosecution anyone who cultivates or uses marijuana on a doctor's recommendation. In the following selection, Linda Peterson tells the story of Dennis Peron, the initiative's controversial spokesperson. She writes that Peron's involvement with medical marijuana began in the late 1980s, when his partner was diagnosed with AIDS and turned to marijuana to combat the severe side effects of his prescription drugs. In 1991, Peron founded San Francisco's Cannabis Buyers Club, which sells marijuana to people with AIDS and other illnesses. However, the author notes, Peron's controversial belief that marijuana should be legalized for nonmedical use has brought him into conflict with both opponents and supporters of the medical marijuana initiative. Peterson is a contributing editor of *Biography*, a monthly entertainment periodical.

As the founding director of San Francisco's Cannabis Buyers Club, Dennis Peron has provided "medical marijuana" to sick people since 1991. Since 1971, he's also sold pot to perfectly healthy citizens, and been convicted for it twice. For his high profile and activism—legal or not—he is a folk hero to many, if not most, residents of his adopted city. "San Francisco loves me," he says, his laugh clear across the telephone line.

Whether or not other Californians feel the same about the man, they agree with his mission: allowing ill people the legal use of pot. Peron was a driving force—some would say the force—behind the controversial Proposition 215, the "medical marijuana initiative," which voters approved in November 1996, 56 to 44 percent. The Compassionate Use Act exempts from prosecution by state authorities anyone who cultivates or uses marijuana on a doctor's recommendation (no prescription is required).

As Peron campaigned for Prop. 215, he had a mantra: "This is more about compassion than marijuana," he would say. "It's time to let doctors decide, not politicians. Stop using patients as pawns!"

A Controversial Advocate

But opponents saw a "stealth" movement whose eventual goal was to legalize marijuana, period—and Peron often made their case as well. He was regularly in the media spotlight, saying things that exasperated even some of his Prop. 215 allies. He'd tell reporters, "I want to be the HMO of marijuana," or "All marijuana use is medical, except for kids." He coauthored a short book entitled *Brownie Mary's Marijuana Cookbook and Dennis Peron's Recipe for Social Change.* "Brownie Mary" Rathbun is 72 and famous for her years of volunteer service baking potlaced brownies for AIDS patients at San Francisco General Hospital. Their book is dedicated to "the 10 million persons who over the past 20 years were arrested for breaking marijuana laws."

And at the Cannabis Buyers Club's election-night celebration, Peron was high on victory—and maybe more. In view of the press, he happily puffed on a joint. (The Prop. 215 triumph likely soothed any disappointment Peron felt at his loss to Bill Clinton: In four states he was also the presidential candidate of the Grass Roots Party.)

Dave Fratello, who promoted Prop. 215 through Californians for Medical Rights (CMR), the Los Angeles base for the initiative, wryly notes that "it wasn't all love" between his camp and Peron's. "The part that became difficult for us was having to take responsibility for the things Dennis said or did," says Fratello. "Dennis didn't want people who were not medical marijuana providers telling him what to do. He likes the spotlight." CMR's media professionals produced commercials aimed at mainstream California voters who, it was feared, might be put off by Peron's image as an "unapologetic pothead," as one article described him.

For his part, says Peron, "I've never shied away from the fact that I think marijuana should have been legalized 25 years ago when Nixon got the recommendation from the Shafer Commission." And from the time the Cannabis Buyers Club opened, he says, they never hid the fact that they were selling marijuana—in baked goods, pills, or smokable forms—to those who presented a doctor's letter of diagnosis saying they had AIDS, cancer, glaucoma, multiple sclerosis, or other conditions for which pot ostensibly provides some relief.

Though selling pot was—and is—a federal offense, top city government and police officials had long adopted a hands-off policy toward the club. But some observers felt that the club's admissions process had become lax: By 1996 there were 12,000 members, some of whom had been accepted with a letter of diagnosis from someone other than a physician—chiropractors, herbalists, even marriage counselors. Some in local law enforcement also charged that Peron was selling to minors, and using dying patients as a cover for a huge drug operation.

They were curious where Peron's own estimate of $200,000 a week in pot sales was going.

Facing a Formidable Foe

Peron's most powerful critic was California Attorney General Dan Lungren, who was also cochairing the "No on 215" lobby. So many saw politics at play when, three months before the 1996 elections, Lungren ordered a raid on Peron's club. On a Sunday morning in August 1996, state narcotics agents wearing riot gear and wielding machine guns seized $60,000 in cash and 150 pounds of pot at the club, and a court order soon shut it down. Lungren's aide at the time said, "The club was running a sophisticated illegal drug distribution network."

The reaction was quirkily San Francisco: The city's mayor, district attorney, sheriff, and police chief all publicly criticized the raid. Stated Mayor Willie Brown, "I am dismayed by the Gestapo tactics displayed by Dan Lungren . . . and wish he would refrain from political grandstanding at the expense of the health and welfare of the people of San Francisco." Fourteen state legislators sent a letter to U.S. Attorney General Janet Reno, charging that Lungren "may have used the power of his office for purely political reasons."

The citizenry was also largely sympathetic: One church even distributed pot to ill people who could prove they were club members. And the criticism went national when cartoonist Garry Trudeau skewered the raid—and Lungren—in his syndicated Doonesbury comic strip.

Nonetheless, CMR's leaders asked Peron to step down as a spokesman for Prop. 215. He refused. Says Dave Fratello, "Let me put it this way: The opposition really wanted Peron to be the initiative's 'poster boy.' Dan Lungren had it very much in mind in making the arrest and promoting it the way they did. They wanted to make Prop. 215 into a referendum on Dennis Peron."

Then three weeks before the election, Peron and five club associates were arrested on felony drug charges. At his arraignment Peron pleaded "morally not guilty." If convicted, he faces life in prison under the state's "three strikes" provision. [In April 2001, Peron pled guilty to misdemeanor conspiracy, but the trial judge dismissed the conviction.]

While declining to discuss the pending criminal case, a spokesman for Lungren said of the timing of the arrests, "That's when the indictment came down."

Answering the Accusations

Peron is defiant. "I'm not worried about it at all, not one little bit," he states. "I'm ready to take them on in court. Lungren tried to paint a picture of me as out of control, selling to minors . . . that never was true, never was proven. We did have four young people come here. All of them had cancer, and their parents' permission.

"As for charges that I'm 'using' sick people—these people are my friends. They're sick and dying, and they need marijuana now—they don't have time to wait for America to make up its mind!" he says heatedly. And in regard to alleged profiteering, Peron has said buying the club's pot supply is incredibly expensive because of the prohibition, and that "every penny" made was plowed back into club operations. (He says the club pays the "astronomical" price of $4,000 to $5,000 a pound for pot.)

"Although I have had a lot of money and a lot of power, I've never, ever used that money or power for my own personal gain," he insists. "I took a vow of poverty in 1967 and I have lived it throughout my life."

He's not keeping up appearances, as it were. Peron drives a faded, ten-year-old van and lives communally in an old Victorian house— "rent controlled," he adds. He owns one suit, worn for events such as legislative appearances. Jokingly referring to himself as a Catholic Buddhist, he maintains that he shares everything in his life. "My grandest possession is my political T-shirt collection," he says with enthusiasm. "I have about 40 shirts dating back to 'LBJ all the way.' If I had to pack something in a fire, that would be it."

Growing Up in New York

Dennis Peron never planned to be a political lightning rod; he wanted to be a psychiatrist. Born in New York's Bronx in 1946, he was raised in a conservative Catholic family, the second of Mary and Albert Peron's five sons. "My father's name actually was Americo because he was the first Italian in his family born here," Dennis says. Now 84, his father worked as an accountant; Mary, of Scottish descent, was a homemaker. At 79, "She's the oldest liver-transplant patient in the world," her son says with pride.

It was his mother, he says, who sparked his compassion for others. "When I was about six, she told me someone was starving in China," he recalls. "She probably said that so I'd eat my lima beans, but I just started to cry. I said, 'Gee, someone's hungry?' From then on I always ate less food. I'm a little guy anyway [five-feet-six, 135 pounds], but to this day I think that if I eat less, there will be more for someone else. I know it's weird, but that's how I think."

The Peron family eventually moved to the Long Island town of Floral Park, where Dennis, the former Cub Scout, took his first puff of pot at age 17. "I didn't get high," he recalls, though in his senior year he says he smoked pot often.

Turning into a Pothead

After graduation he enrolled in the local community college and began taking psychology courses. But when he took a semester off, he got a draft notice. He chose to sign up with the Air Force, somehow believing he would avoid Vietnam. Considering his counterculture image today, it seems logical to ask: Why didn't he run off to Canada?

"I was a pretty straight kid," he replies. "Though in hindsight, I think I just wanted to get out of my dreadful old town." In 1967 he was sent to Vietnam. During the Tet offensive, one of his duties was retrieving the bodies of American soldiers. "Vietnam was hell . . . it turned me into a pothead," he says. Bullets whizzing by him also had another effect. "I was tired of suppressing these feelings I was having, and I just came out of the closet, to find my identity as a gay man."

He adds, "When I told my mom I had a boyfriend, her first question was, 'Is he Catholic?' I said 'Ma, what does it matter—we're not going to have babies! But we do have a poodle.'"

After the military, Peron settled in San Francisco and into his activism: gay rights, civil rights, hippie causes, any effort to legalize marijuana. He had flown back from Vietnam with two pounds of pot, and began selling it "to make ends meet" while he enrolled at the city college to study psychiatry. "Every time I'd sell a bag I'd talk to the people about their problems," he relates. "I realized that people were using this as medicine, for stress reduction or depression . . . and I thought, hey, I am sort of a psychiatrist!"

Dealing overtook studying. In the mid-'70s Peron ran a "pot supermarket" and a vegetarian restaurant downstairs from it. Ever the activist, he had an unorthodox method for encouraging civic duty: "I forced my customers to register to vote before I would sell them pot."

Over the years he racked up 15 arrests, two convictions, and spent two years in jail.

The Birth of an Activist

Peron's transition from "genial street scoundrel," as one writer called him, to a man on a mission occurred in 1988—when his partner of seven years, artist Jonathan West, was diagnosed with AIDS. (Peron is HIV-negative.) On a 24-hour basis Peron watched the man suffer severe side effects from the "dozens of prescription drugs" he was taking. "The one drug that stopped his nausea when he got cancer treatment, eased his pain, and restored his appetite, was marijuana," he recalls. "It worked such wonders for him, and I thought, this is such a utilitarian drug!" In 1990, West testified at Peron's latest trial for drug possession, telling the court that the pot found in the apartment had been his medicine. The charges against Peron were dropped. West died two weeks later. "When Jonathan died, I dedicated my life to this cause as his legacy," says Peron.

In 1991, Peron spearheaded a city initiative to allow the medical use of pot—it passed with a 79-percent approval rate. With that support, he opened the Buyers Club, now housed in a five-story office building near City Hall. Statewide, he worked for two medical marijuana bills that passed the State Legislature with bipartisan support, but were then vetoed by Governor Pete Wilson.

At that point, Peron and others decided to "take it to the people" with a veto proof ballot initiative. He sought out a more mainstream cosponsor: Anna Boyce, a 67-year-old senior assembly woman whom he'd met when they both testified for previous bills. Boyce, a resident of conservative Orange County and a registered nurse, had illegally obtained pot for her husband, John, when he was dying of cancer.

"It took me a solid month to convince him to try it because he was concerned about the disgrace," Boyce recalls. "But he took two puffs—and he stopped vomiting. He looked at me and said, 'I don't feel sick. You got something to eat?' He had lost 30 pounds, but he put every bit back on by the time he died [six months later]."

She and Peron set about writing Prop. 215. "He had ideas, I had ideas. We wanted to make it broad enough to cover anyone." Of the common criticism that the measure has no age restriction, she replies, "Children do develop cancer and AIDS. The child doesn't make the decision [to use pot]—the doctor knows when nothing else is working. And the child doesn't have to smoke it, you know; it can be put in butter and spread on vegetables." And though Boyce disapproves of legalizing pot for nonmedicinal use, she does approve of Dennis.

In November 1996, the voters agreed. In January 1997, so did the city judge who ordered that Peron's club be allowed to reopen. The judge cited "the will of the people," as evidenced by the Prop. 215 victory.

Life After Victory

For now, Dennis Peron is back to his routine at the renamed Cannabis Cultivators Club. About 3000 members have registered, and perhaps 300 visit on a given day. "I try to greet and talk with everyone who comes in," says Peron. The club is growing its first crop of marijuana inside the building, but still must "contract" with large growers for the bulk of its supply. Peron says it's critically important to provide a product without the molds or pesticides that can cause respiratory infections, potentially deadly to someone with AIDS.

All members come for the pot; many stay for socializing and support groups. "We have a 12-step drug program that includes marijuana as part of its therapy," explains Peron. "You know, people keep saying marijuana use is a gateway, gateway, gateway—but marijuana is a gateway out of alcoholism, out of crack and meth [amphetamine] addiction. It's one hope they can get off it."

He concedes marijuana is not without health hazards, and shouldn't normally be used by anyone under 18, but insists that the government's drug policies are misdirected.

"There is a pecking order [of drug danger], and marijuana is not the one that should be pecked," he states. "Let the government peck on alcohol and tobacco, and methamphetamine and crack and heroin—the drugs that are killing people!" As for himself, Peron says he gave up drinking in 1980, but admits he's "addicted to cigarettes."

Peron and others also like to point out what they see as the ultimate hypocrisy in the federal war on pot: Since 1976, the U.S. Food and Drug Administration has operated a "compassionate use" experimental drug program that legally provides free marijuana to eight Americans, whose medical conditions include cancer, multiple sclerosis, genetic disease, and glaucoma. The program closed to new patients in 1992.

Whatever legal troubles lie ahead, Peron says his focus remains clear. "I'm just seeing this thing through," he says. "I'm doing it so that we will become a more compassionate country. I'm doing it for Jonathan and all the young people who have died of AIDS. So the critics can say anything they want about me. I really don't care."

Marijuana Entrepreneurs

Jake MacDonald

In the following selection, Jake MacDonald takes a look at the booming marijuana business in Vancouver, Canada. He profiles several entrepreneurs in various facets of the marijuana trade, as well as law enforcement officers whose job is to prevent marijuana smuggling. Although marijuana is not legal, the author writes, the penalties for possession are small, and the economic rewards have led people from all walks of life to grow and sell marijuana. MacDonald also describes the challenges of growing marijuana: For example, since 90 percent of the marijuana produced in Vancouver is grown indoors under artificial light, the enormous consumption of electricity that is required often draws the attention of law enforcement. Those who smuggle the marijuana crop into the United States confront the greatest risk, MacDonald explains, facing the possibility of long prison sentences in U.S. jails if they are caught. MacDonald is a writer and contributing editor for magazines such as *Chatelaine*, *Canadian Geographic*, and *Saturday Night*.

It's 2 A.M. in Vancouver, drizzling rain, and a faint blue television light is burning in a sixth-floor window of the Sylvia Hotel. Inside the room, a thirty-nine-year-old bachelor we'll call Ryan is lying on a double bed, rolling a number and watching *The Wild Bunch* on the movie channel. It's a well-made movie, but director Sam Peckinpah's tale of an aging gang's final bid for riches has too much gunfire and mayhem for Ryan's deliberative mood. So he thumbs the remote and flits through the channels, pondering the complex architecture of his next move.

At six feet tall and 200 pounds, Ryan is a handsome, lazy-dog sort of man, with a good collection of novels in his duffle bag and a wry comment always on the tip of his tongue. In one of these late movies, he'd be the good-natured cowboy who also robs banks. After growing up as a commercial pilot's son in northern Ontario, Ryan roamed all over Canada and worked at a variety of jobs—bartender, newspaper reporter, ski instructor—before landing here in Vancouver. He has an easy life now, with few responsibilities, no kids, no home. But he still feels a weight gathering on him. He'll be forty soon, and has a spooky vision of himself five years from now, still drinking beer with a bunch of morons at the Marble Arch. Swinging out of bed, he blows smoke out the window, and surveys the distant lights of the freighters anchored in English Bay. "Tomorrow," he says, "I'll show you the sailboat I want to buy. I'm going to take about eighteen months and explore my way down the coast of Mexico. Go through the Panama Canal, and then up through the Caribbean. Eventually I'll run a charter business out of Grand Bahama or Bimini. I've been planning it for about ten years, and it's time to go."

The Invisible Economy

He's done the research, talked to sailing veterans, and figures he needs about $200,000 to buy the boat and finance the move. He doesn't want a loan. He'll export a few loads of marijuana to the United States. He's been dabbling in the marijuana business for the last couple of years anyway, owning pieces of various operations around the city, and he's decided that it's time to get serious. "You can make a fast two or three hundred thousand without much trouble," he says. "We're producing the best weed in the world. We're exporting hundreds of tons of the stuff, but the Americans still want more."

Tossing his roach into the night, Ryan surveys the few windows that are still aglow in the apartment building across the street. "You look out at the city, I bet there's a dozen grow operations within sight of this window. It's Vancouver's invisible economy."

In 1989, you could have symbolized the red-blooded British Columbia resource sector with a photograph of a commercial fisherman and a hog-fat chinook salmon. But now the salmon has turned into a bale of marijuana. Police estimate that the annual British Columbia marijuana crop is worth about $2 billion. Marijuana activists say it's larger, but nobody disputes that dope growing has become a mammoth resource industry in B.C., worth at least twice as much as all the wholesale fisheries revenues combined.

Marijuana is traditionally an outdoor crop. But in the late 1980s, B.C. marijuana growers began experimenting with hydroponic systems, in which plants are grown indoors, without soil, in a mixture of nutrient-rich water and rock pellets. Nowadays, about 90 percent of British Columbia's crop is grown indoors. "You don't have to worry about bugs, animals, rip-off artists, and police helicopters," says Ryan. "And because you supply the perfect mix of nutrients and light, you get a higher yield." In a hydroponic operation, each plant produces about half a pound of usable marijuana. The crop is sold for about $3,000 per pound to middlemen, who then break it down into smaller bags and sell it to their friends and neighbours, or stockpile it for export to the United States. Methods used for smuggling are limited only by the imagination. In magazines like *High Times* and *Cannabis Culture* there are accounts of smugglers using hollowed-out drift logs, dead whales, and remote-controlled midget submarines to export their weed across the strait that separates B.C. from Washington. But in reality, most of the crop probably moves south in more mundane ways: via fishing boats, semi-trailers, private cars, pickups, bicycles, or even by foot, using "mules"—human couriers who haul it across in backpacks. "The couriers are the ones you feel sorry for," says Sergeant Pete Thompson of the Royal Canadian Mounted Police (RCMP) detachment at Chilliwack. "They're often people who are down on their luck and desperate to make some quick money. They get paid a couple of thousand dollars in return for a night's work. But when they get caught, they're in an awful lot of trouble."

Nobody knows how much marijuana is flowing across the border into the United States, but law enforcement authorities estimate that they intercept only about one percent of the traffic. "Most of the marijuana in the southwestern United States still comes from Mexico," says Dave Keller, an intelligence agent with the United States Border Patrol based in Blaine, Washington, just south of Vancouver. "But your B.C. bud is so popular in California that we've had a tremendous increase in seizures over the last couple of years." Even so, the 500-kilometre-long boundary between British Columbia and Washington is so lightly patrolled, according to Keller, that smugglers tend to regard it as "no more than a minor inconvenience."

Preparing for a Border Crossing

Last week Ryan cancelled the lease on his apartment. Yesterday he broke up with his girlfriend. Now he's speeding around Vancouver in a twenty-eight-year-old sports car with sheepskin seat covers, a walnut shifter knob, and a good selection of Lou Reed tapes in the glovebox, burning bridges behind him. He likes to drive "up on the torque curve," which means that the car is always lunging forward or decelerating wildly, and accompanying him for a drive around town is a physical workout.

When you consider Ryan's flamboyant car, his disdain for traffic flow, and the fact that he needs a clean record for his upcoming border crossings, you'd expect him to think twice before roaring around with a baggie of ganja in plain view on the dashboard. But in Vancouver, the paranoid sixties are truly over. "Simple possession is basically legal," says Ryan. "If the cop's in a bad mood, he might tell you to empty it on the road."

Anyway, Ryan is a busy man, and traffic cops are the least of his worries. He's gearing up for battle with bigger dragons, the ones that guard the American border. He figures he can either skirt around them, by slipping across the darkened border on foot, by boat, or by kayak, or he can just throw forty pounds of marijuana in his car and meet them head-on. He's considering all the options, running his own feasibility study.

"A few days ago I made a test run," he says. "As a mental exercise I strapped a hockey bag to the luggage rack. When I pulled up to U.S. Customs they just waved me through. But then I noticed I was being followed by a blue van with beacons on the roof. I slowed down, it slowed down. I turned down a dirt road, and it followed me. Finally I pulled over, and the van stopped, two feet behind me. By now, I'm sweating, even though there's nothing in the bag but laundry. This guy in a uniform gets out, walks towards me, and puts a bundle of letters into a mailbox. It's the U.S. Postal Service."

Ryan comes to a screeching halt in the parking lot of a Vancouver marina. He wants to inspect a prospective sailboat—a thirty-six-foot sloop with ocean-going navigational equipment, gleaming brass hardware, and a mahogany-panelled stateroom with seven feet of headroom. The vendor has slyly left a Jimmy Buffet tape in the sound system, and the music plays softly while Ryan quibbles with the broker. It's a glorious day in Vancouver, banner-blue sky, buzzing seaplanes, and a distant backdrop of snow-capped mountains. Sitting on the fantail, I'm visualizing the turquoise tidal flats of the Bahamas, the palm trees waving at the harbour entrance to Freeport, and wondering if Ryan will actually ever make it there. By his own confession, he's a seasoned procrastinator, and this could be just another Jimmy Buffet daydream—or what Ryan calls "pot brain-lock." Ryan smokes marijuana regularly, but admits there are drawbacks. "Pot brain-lock is when you get a great idea," he explains. "Then you can't remember what it was."

For the last couple of years, Ryan has been helping people set up grow operations in their basements. He installs the plumbing, wiring, and exhaust conduits, and in return takes a share of the profits. He says marijuana growers have two options when they're launching a new operation—they can start from scratch with seeds, or they can grow their plants from cuttings. Seeds can produce either male or female plants, so half the crop will inevitably be thrown away (only female plants produce enough tetrahydrocannabinol (THC) to get you high); and they have to be germinated, a time-consuming process. "Seeds are for rookies," Ryan says. They do, however, afford an easy and quasi-legal entryway into the business. A novice like me couldn't just walk into a store in Vancouver and buy a lush, mature, female marijuana plant. He could, however, buy seeds.

Talking with Marijuana Shop Owners

Downtown, Ryan squeezes his car into a narrow spot just down the hill from the Amsterdam Hemporium Coffee Shop, a place that typifies British Columbia's tentative drift towards marijuana legalization. When we walk in the door, jazz is playing softly from speakers in the ceiling, and the skunky odour of marijuana is drifting on the air. We order coffee and carrot cake and peruse the wall by our table, where a montage of photographs shows scenes from the Cannabis Cup—an international marijuana trade show held annually in Amsterdam. The shop's proprietors, Sita von Windheim and Karen Watson, figure prominently in the montage. Both are photogenic and, judging from the evidence, numerous glassy-eyed Cannabis Cup delegates were eager to pose at their side. But when they join us, they seem to be no-nonsense entrepreneurs, with the same headaches and ambitions as any other shop owners. "I rarely even smoke it," says Sita, a fashionable brunette with a large, diamond-studded ring on her hand. "I'm a single mother with three kids, and frankly, I don't have the time."

Karen Watson, Sita's thirty-year-old business partner, has straight blonde hair and the perky, wholesome demeanour of a California surfer. After graduating from the University of British Columbia (UBC) with a Bachelor of Science degree, she joined forces with Sita and opened the shop in 1997. Pulling up a chair, Karen opens her catalogue and spreads some marijuana seeds on the table. "We've been charged by the police for selling these," she says. "But the case hasn't gone to court, so it's not exactly clear to us whether the seeds themselves are illegal." Their catalogue advertises 150 hybrids of two basic types of marijuana: *indica*, a plant that favours more temperate climates and is reputed to induce a somewhat physical, dopey high; and *sativa*, a tropical strain with a lighter, more cerebral effect. When Bill Clinton fired up a joint back in the 1960s, the marijuana that he didn't inhale was almost certainly *sativa*. Historically, the world's largest marijuana exporters have been sativa-producing countries like Mexico and Jamaica. British Columbia's recent dominance in the field is partially due to the high quality of its *indica* marijuana. "We may not be producing the best in the world," says Karen, who studied the physiology of narcotics at UBC, "but it's the best in North America."

I tell her about a Vancouver grower who told me that he has a "mother plant" hybridized by botanists working for the Hell's Angels that is worth $15,000 as breeding stock. "Marijuana growers are like fishermen," Karen replies. "They're somewhat prone to exaggeration."

Flipping through their catalogue, she points out the range of choices. The seeds run from first-class, expensive varieties like "Northern Lights" ("dominates the Harvest Festivals—the most powerful plant in the world—$300.00 for 10 seeds") to cheaper, hardier outdoor varieties like "Fast Manitoba" ("grows to 4–5 feet and yields a quarter pound. $40 for 10 seeds"). Sita and Karen say that they have an 80 percent germination rate for all of the seeds in their catalogue, as long as they are babied in accordance with the instructions. With a smile, Karen adds, "We don't, however, encourage anyone to act in conflict with the law."

Ryan laughs. There are a dozen customers in the restaurant, most of them college kids in baggy flannel shirts and khakis. They're drinking tea, rolling joints, and puffing on pipes stuffed with marijuana. "If they break the law, it's not our responsibility," Sita insists. "But I don't think there's anything wrong with what they're doing. Kids are going to smoke pot. And I'd rather my daughters did that than drink alcohol. It's less toxic."

Karen nods. "The fact is, dopers are nice people. And countless medical studies have proved that marijuana is harmless. Why should it be against the law?"

"Well, I can think of one reason," says Ryan, zipping up his jacket as we head down the hill to the car. "If they legalized it, the bottom would fall out of the market. Then how would I buy my sailboat?"

The Attitude of Law Enforcement

Police say there are thousands of grow houses in the Vancouver area, so many that they don't even bother to look for them. "We don't have to," says Corporal Brian Cantera of the Langley detachment of the RCMP. "We have more than we can deal with already."

Cantera says the public has the impression that the RCMP have decided on their own to fight the marijuana industry. "That's not how it works," he says. "We don't go around looking for boarded-up houses, saying, 'Oh look, those people are growing marijuana. Let's arrest them.' There's a very strong feeling in Langley that large-scale marijuana growing is a serious social problem. People are very upset about it. We have town hall meetings, landlords who are angry because the growers rent their houses and then cut big holes in the walls and start electrical fires. People see this as a threat to their community. They're the ones who are asking the RCMP to make it a priority."

The stereotype of the drug dealer—the young, anti-social male with a poor employment history and a criminal record—no longer applies to the typical Vancouver pot grower, "We get every type of person you can imagine," says RCMP investigator Dave Duplissie. "I can't emphasize that too much. There's no typical offender. We get people with clean records, middle-class professionals, nice elderly people, retired couples, Asian immigrants, you name it." Marijuana is becoming as socially acceptable as alcohol in B.C., and the high rewards and minimal penalties associated with growing it have lured individuals from every level of society.

Some prosecutors have been asking for stiffer penalties for marijuana growers. But according to a prominent Vancouver-area lawyer, John Conroy, the courts are moving in the opposite direction. "Recent federal legislation says that we should be looking at alternatives to imprisonment. For medium-sized cultivation cases—say a hundred plants—courts usually impose a fine of several thousand dollars. Many growers regard this as a simple cost of doing business."

But marijuana cultivation is still an "indictable offence," which means convicted offenders have to admit to their crimes on job applications, and will be barred from entering the United States for the rest of their lives. Growers therefore are a secretive lot, and hard to find. I keep pushing Ryan to find me a grow room, and one evening he wangles us a dinner invitation from a young couple—a double-income family with a five-year-old son and a whopping mortgage. They live in a plush neighbourhood near Marine Drive. He's a civil servant; she's an advertising executive. Ryan met them through mutual friends, and for a third of the action, he manages the technical side of their small hydroponic operation. The family uses the profits to defray the costs of living in Vancouver. "Tell them you're writing about the marijuana business," Ryan advises me. "But don't say any more than that."

During dinner my hosts offer helpful advice. "How about this?" the lady of the house keeps remarking. "I know somebody who used to grow pot in Kelowna. Would you like her phone number?" After dinner, we retire to the living room, sip an expensive imported beer, and discuss further leads that might be helpful to my research. They never once mention the grow operation in their basement.

The next day I make an appointment to see a man who refers to himself as Professor Puff. Like a dozen or so other equipment suppliers in the city, he's listed in the Yellow Pages and offers technical advice to people who want to start hydroponic operations in their homes. "What I do is totally legal," he says. "We just give advice and sell equipment. What you do with it when you get home is your business."

With his denim-bib coveralls, ponytail, and drooping outlaw-biker moustache, Puff is about as mild-mannered as you can be and still look like security at a Rolling Stones concert. His cluttered shop is stacked to the ceiling with big, bulbous metal-halide lights, plastic conduit, and exotic liquid fertilizers. Pouring himself a coffee, he flips open a notebook. "Before we get started, I'm going to ask you something. Are you ready for a commitment of one hour a day? If you're going to grow these little plants, you have to accept that you're going to be their daddy." I make a note of it.

"One hour a day," he insists. "Every day. No more two-week vacations. You wouldn't do it to your pet, and you can't do it to your plants." Punching the button on his ballpoint, he writes down a list of materials. "Now—we base everything on the size of your rooms. How big are your growing rooms?"

"Let's say two small, eight-by-ten bedrooms."

"Do you want to grow the plants in pots of dirt or in hydroponic solution?"

"What's easier?"

"Dirt. It's more forgiving."

"Dirt it is." On a piece of paper, he draws two rectangles and a rough floor plan. "You're looking at about three thousand dollars' worth of equipment for two basic rooms. The first room is the veg room where you keep eight mother plants. They're mature females, and you never harvest them. They're for cuttings. You hang two big metal-halide lights above the mothers, rigged to a timer. Eighteen hours of daylight, and six of dark. To get started, you take fifty or sixty cuttings off the mothers and start them in little grow trays."

I write it all down. "Where do I get my mothers?"

"You grow them from seeds that you buy from suppliers like Karen Watson and Sita von Windheim, over at the Amsterdam cafe. Or you start them from cuttings."

Learning to Grow a Marijuana Crop

His cellular phone keeps ringing, but he ignores it. "Your fifty or sixty cuttings are like a litter of puppies. After six weeks, you pick out twenty-four of the happiest ones and move them into the other room."

"What do you do with the runts?"

"Whatever you like. They make great little presents. Marijuana is a beautiful plant, whether you smoke it or not. Everybody should have one."

"What's next?"

"The other room is called the bloom room." Scribbling with his pen, he sketches in six lights, spaced equidistantly across the room. The plants are arranged below, four plants per light. "Set your timer for twelve hours of HID—that's high in density discharge light—and twelve of darkness. When the lights are on, plants inhale carbon dioxide and exhale oxygen. Thank God for them, or there'd be no life on earth. In the darkness, they do the opposite. We install a CO_2 generator on the floor, set it for about fifteen-hundred parts per million, and pump the used air out of the room with an exhaust system."

"Vent the exhaust out into the yard?"

"Yep. But to get rid of the smell, you install an ozonator on the exhaust pipe."

"What's an ozonator?"

"It's basically an ultraviolet light that's ten times stronger than a tanning lamp. Any odour molecule going by gets cleaned and scrubbed. Out in the yard, you can't smell a thing."

He hands me the sketches of the two floor plans. "You want to keep the temperature variation in the room at no more than ten degrees. Put two oscillating fans in each corner of the room. They keep the room cool, and make the plants healthy and strong. Once you're up and running, you should be able to harvest twenty-four plants every six weeks."

"And what's a harvest like that worth, wholesale?"

"Twelve thousand, minimum."

"So people are making a lot of money at this?"

"Most people end up losing their asses."

"Why?"

"Same reason as always. They get busted by the cops."

"How?"

"Same reason as always. They're idiots."

The Cost of Doing Business

"I think of fines as my GST [Goods and Services Tax]," says Glenn, a slender, clean-cut thirty-eight-year-old with a taste for leather Stetson hats and vegetarian cooking. In 1993, Glenn, who prefers not to use his real name, was an electrician with the B.C. government. He moved in with a buddy, and discovered that his roommate was making an extra $100,000 a year growing marijuana. "I sort of learned the business from him," he says. When the government offered Glenn a severance package, he took it and went into marijuana cultivation full time. He's been doing it now for five years, and makes about $13,000 per month. "I'm very small time," he says. "Thousands of people in Vancouver are running bigger shows. But I do it because I love the job, the science and the art of gardening. The technology is always evolving, and if you're into that, like I am, there's a lot of satisfaction in perfecting your operation."

Glenn now lives in an expensive home in south Vancouver, and tonight, Ryan and I have dropped over to see his operation. He's been arrested twice, he tells us. The first time, he was speeding down the highway in his Grand Wagoneer, delivering a couple of pounds of freshly harvested bud. He was speeding because he was tense about missing the ferry, and smoking a bomber because he was tense. When the RCMP officer pulled him over, she almost had to fan the smoke away with her hat.

The second time, he says, "some crazy crackhead" broke into his house, discovered his grow room in the basement, and confessed his discovery to the cops in return for undisclosed favours. Glenn's neighbour, who apparently has connections with the police department, dropped over and warned Glenn that his name was on the hit list. "I got rid of most of my plants," Glenn says. "But I had these six lovely mothers, and I just couldn't stand to part with them." A few days later, the cops came through the door like the Pittsburgh Steelers. "They were shouting, waving guns, the whole thing. I grow herbs for my kitchen, and one of them got excited when he saw all those little plants. I told him they were just herbs, and he was disgusted. 'Look, the guys a regular Martha Stewart.' They took my six marijuana plants. But I think they were so disappointed with their haul that they never came back."

His cases haven't gone to court yet, but if he's found guilty, he believes he'll get a $500 fine for the first offence and $1,500 for the second. He brokered a dope deal today and made $6,000 in a couple of hours. So fines of that size are not much of a concern. Still, there's a nervous twitch in his smile as he tells me about his arrest record. "I can't afford to get busted again. They might send me to jail."

Located in a sealed-off room in his basement, Glenn's operation is evocative of those seriously eccentric bait shops you find in lake country—the odd smell, the treacherous stairs leading down into the gloomy cellar, the bewildering maze of wires, the gurgling pipes, the secret room, and then, under a ferocious bath of light—the little monsters. Buffeted by two oscillating fans, they ripple and preen their leaves as if alive. Glenn seems almost ready to apologize to them for walking into the room unannounced. He nods toward a tape deck on the table. "They really enjoy the Three Tenors."

Glenn's plants are just beginning to produce the buds that will soon be resinous, purplish clumps of blossoms about the size of a child's fist. He estimates that his crop will be worth about $90,000 if it's sold in San Francisco. "If you took it to Hawaii," says Ryan, "you could double that amount."

Waiting for Customers

The lights in Glenn's grow room are painfully brilliant, and it's a relief to go back upstairs. Tonight, two Californians are coming over to talk business, and Ryan, who smells American currency, wants to meet them. The buyers are late, so up in the kitchen, Glenn pours glasses of red wine and lapses into a nagging debate with Ryan about electrical wiring. Marijuana growers face one intractable problem—hydro consumption. An average household might consume 1,500 kilowatts per month. A small operation like Glenn's will push the monthly draw up to about 4,000 kilowatts. Anything larger is likely to attract attention from the police. One drug officer told me, "We can't go into a house just because of somebody's hydro bill, but we use it as a strong piece of evidence when we're approaching the court for a search warrant." Rural growers often use generators, and in one recent case the RCMP uncovered an ingenious grow operation inside a buried school bus, with hidden wiring, and exhaust vents from the bus exiting into above-ground trash barrels. In the city, growers are stuck with using power from the hydro grid, and it makes them nervous.

Glenn says he has a friend who fools the meter by dismantling it halfway through the month, flipping the wheel over and letting it run backwards for a week. Every meter has a seal on it to foil tampering, but his friend has a connection who gives him boxes of fresh seals. "My own hydro bill is still about three hundred dollars a month. But this neighbourhood has lots of hot tubs and swimming pools, so I probably blend in."

Ryan says he's seen grow houses where the wheel in the meter spins so quickly you could sharpen your skates on it. "The cops are like sub hunters," he says. "We're throwing off a ping, ping, they're closing in, and there's not much we can do about it."

I ask Glenn about these buyers of his. After all, he barely knows them. What if they walk in the door and put a gun in his face? "It's not like the movies," he says. "It's really low-key. We listen to a bit of music, smoke some bud. Talk about wilderness camping or whatever. We do the switch, they give me the money. I don't even count it. They're pretty nice people in the pot business."

They may be nice people but they're not much at timetables. Apparently they've already missed two appointments with Glenn this week, and now they're several hours late. "Pot brain-lock," sniffs Ryan, as we head out the door.

Visiting the Smuggling Routes

Two days later, I rise at two-thirty in the morning and cruise out through the deserted streets of Vancouver. In an hour, I'm at the Aldergrove crossing, a port of entry into the United States. Light rain is misting down through the mercury-vapour lamps above the parking lot. The office windows of U.S. Customs are dark, and the checkpoint booths are empty.

Everyone is home in bed. At this hour, even local police detachments are closed, or operating with a single car for emergencies. For a few minutes I sit there with the wipers clapping, looking at the empty road, imagining that I'm Ryan and I've got a duffle bag with forty pounds of marijuana in the trunk. What's to stop me from just driving through? Probably there's a video camera connected to a sleepy control room somewhere. But on the Washington side there's a maze of back roads. And when the cop finally arrives, he'll be searching for a needle in a haystack. Fourteen hours from now, I could be sitting in a fancy restaurant in San Francisco, having just bundled $240,000 into my Bank of America safety-deposit box.

Turning right, I drive west along a deserted secondary road. It's dark, with an occasional gleam in the distance to mark a farmer's yard light. This is Zero Avenue. If I stopped the car and took two steps, I'd be in the United States. The fields are studded with head-high trellises for the raspberry crop, and here and there in the ditch, you can see tire tracks where smugglers have simply doused their headlights and driven south between the rows. If I were Ryan, I'd try to avoid the video camera at the port of entry and just drive through the field. I'd never suspect that a dozen men in fatigues are crouched in the darkness, waiting for me.

A kilometre west of here, an enormous camera sits atop a tall tripod, aimed along the border. The cable leads to the tailgate of a truck, where two men are watching the monitor. Dave Keller of the U.S. Border Patrol is there, dressed in green raingear. The man beside him, in dark blue RCMP coveralls, is Pete Thompson. The big infrared camera reveals a gelled, greenish world, alive with ghosts. In the distance, a farm truck creeps along Zero Avenue, its undercarriage pulsing like neon in the viewer. A while later a wraith-like pheasant sneaks across the road, followed by the shadowy heat signature of a fox. I can hear portable radios crackle as other officers report in. The Mounties are watching potential getaway routes to the north in unmarked cars. American Border Patrol officers are hiding in the fields to the south in waterproof fatigues. They're spread out along ten kilometres of border.

Catching Smugglers

A single organization, the Integrated Border Enforcement Team, or IBET, has brought Keller and Thompson together tonight. IBET was masterminded by Thompson, and after the team became operational in 1998, they ran a campaign called *Eh, Quo Vadis?* (Where do you think you're going, eh?), and started catching marijuana smugglers and other traffickers right away: Thompson's storage room in Chilliwack is stacked to the ceiling with pungent sacks of marijuana and other contraband. Thompson has chosen this godforsaken place because it's the last place a smuggler would expect to find him. "We'll see some action," he says. "I guarantee it."

We crouch behind the tailgate in the freezing rain watching the monitor. We can hear the yelp of geese drifting down from the overcast. "Most of this country is farmland," Dave Keller says, "miles of dirt road, woods, swamp. We've got motion sensors here and there, but they're not always reliable. This rainy climate is hell on equipment. We get gunrunners, suspected terrorists, and undocumented aliens coming through as well. If there are any marijuana smugglers out there tonight, they might pull up in a truck, toss the stuff over a fence into Washington, then call their contacts with a cell phone."

Thompson locates the IBET stakeouts in apparently random fashion, trying to anticipate the routes the smugglers will be using. "Sometimes it works almost too well," he says. "One night I flashed my headlights, and a smuggler ran across the border and jumped in my truck. Just about everybody on the team has had that happen."

"We get a pretty good class of smuggler around here," Keller says. "They use radio scanners, night-vision goggles. They watch us, just like we watch them."

The radio crackles. One of the Mounties is calling in from his hiding place to report that a pickup truck with yellow running lights on the roof has just passed him, moving slowly. Soon it becomes visible on the monitor, creeping along Zero Avenue, its chassis aglow. And even though it's cold and wet here in the field, I'm glad I'm not the guy driving the truck.

It stops, almost on cue, about a kilometre away from us. On the monitor, two glowing human silhouettes roll out and gallop south into the raspberry field. Thompson barks an order and the radio begins to boil over with the chaotic sounds of pursuit—slamming doors, gunning engines, unintelligible shouting over the static, and the confused cries of men chasing the runners on foot.

If Ryan is unlucky, this is how his dream will end. Instead of lazing on his yacht in the Caribbean, he'll find himself gum-booting through a muddy field with a dozen cops on his tail and a U.S. jail sentence in his future. The last time I talked with him, we were sitting on a park bench in the sun, by the waterfront, watching the cyclists glide by. He'd drifted west all his life, but now the ocean was only a stone's throw away, and as far as he was concerned, there was no place left to go. He didn't know when or how he was going to take a load across, but his mind seemed made up. "Maybe at one time, I could have had a normal life. I could have gotten married, raised some kids. But it's a seductive thing, the marijuana business. You get used to the money, and you can sleep in whenever you want. Then one day you realize that you've turned into Smiley [a fictional spy]. And it's too late to come in from the cold."

FIGHTING AMERICA'S WAR ON MARIJUANA

Steve White, interviewed by Elena Mannes

Steve White is a former agent for the Drug Enforcement Agency who for five years led Indiana's war on marijuana. In the following selection, *Frontline* producer Elena Mannes interviews White concerning his experiences with marijuana growers and his opinions about the dangers of marijuana. White confesses that, contrary to his expectations, most growers involved in the illegal marijuana business turned out to be normal Americans rather than violent criminals. Nevertheless, he contends that these growers are still knowingly engaged in illegal activities and should be punished appropriately. Although some people argue that marijuana is not as dangerous as other drugs and therefore the penalties should be more lenient, White points out that he has seen families and lives ruined because of marijuana. White is currently an instructor of undercover police techniques.

Elena Mannes: Can you talk about the growers you have met over the years?
   Steve White: Twenty years before I had done a lot of undercover work—it was mainly amphetamine, LSD, heroin and cocaine—I thought all the dealers were scum. When I got into the marijuana program, one thing that amazed me was how cooperative a lot of the people were. How proud of what they're doing. How normal in every other respect they were.

A Different Kind of Lawbreaker

This is confusing and I'm not used to lawbreakers that took their kids to school and worked as crossing guards and that sort of thing. Whole different attitude. It made it a lot more complex, but it made it a lot more interesting.

   Then, as I learned more about the agriculture, itself, and was able to talk to these people, they became even more interesting because they had devoted a lot of time into learning as much as they could. The amount of expertise that they had was at the university level quite a bit because I went to IU [Indiana University] and talked to

From *Frontline*'s Report "Busted: America's War on Marijuana," a Steve White interview by Elena Mannes, April 28, 1998. www.pbs.org/frontline/shows/dope. Used with permission.

people in the biology department to find out what was being done.

They were always on the cutting edge of the technology and they took some very common technology and utilized it in the growers. So, I'd have to honestly say I was impressed by them and I found a lot of them to be engaging personally. There's some of them that I, quite frankly, like. But I still put 'em in jail. They're breaking the law.

But they're different. They're not crack dealers. They're not South Americans with machine guns. But here, thank goodness, we were able to escape the violence in some other areas. I think part of it was the philosophy of law enforcement here in Indiana. We did not go up and crash through doors. You cannot flush down 300 pounds of marijuana and 15 growing lights and the attendant equipment.

We'd walk up and knock on the door. Here we are. Let you do it peacefully, and most of the time we go in with a video camera and they'd take us through and tell us where, because there are danger areas in there as far as electric power and water and fertilizers, and most of them cooperated, which I wasn't used to. I can't recall one ever physically resisting. Sometimes they're a little unhappy, and there was harsh language used, but that doesn't hurt.

So they're different. They impress me.

Drawing Conclusions

Did you come to any conclusions?

I still reflect about it. We've got alcohol, we've got tobacco. Why are so many people dedicated to this drug? I don't believe it has any medicinal value. At one time, the government did run a program, which I partially administered here, where we had marijuana cigarettes available. We couldn't find a physician in the state that would write a prescription for them. It's been much ballyhooed, but that existed for over ten years and the medical community rejected it.

I think a lot of people that grow, actually grow it to stay off the mean streets. They don't have to go out and buy dope, and go to the places where it's sold and deal with the people that sell it. But the downside and reverse side of that is sometime along the line they say, "Gee, I've spent this much on equipment and this much on fertilizer. Why don't I grow a little more and sell it, and pay for that?"

People get hurt, not physically, but families get hurt. It happens, but that's very fair and simple. If you're in there, in your house, growing marijuana for your own use, chances are we will probably never show up, because you're not going to use that much power. Nothing, people are not going to know about it. You asked me about informants. One year, we did three indoor grows here based on the children [of] the growers, through the D.A.R.E. [Drug Abuse Resistance Education] program. They not only told us about it. They drew diagrams. How to get to daddy's indoor grow. So, that's tough on a family.

Well, if the law is creating a situation in which kids are spying on their parents. Do you think about that?

Oh, I don't see that like Nazi Germany or Communist Russia. No. No. I just put that out because it happened and I find that unusual, noteworthy, maybe even scary. But on the other hand, most people in this country will tell you they want education on drug abuse. This is what you're going to get from your educator.

Marijuana Should Be Illegal

What do you think about the idea of decriminalization?

I am just opposed to decriminalizing it. Where do we stop? Do we tell our young people that marijuana's bad, but under 30 grams is good? That doesn't make sense. If 30 grams is good, then 31 grams, what's bad about that? They're intelligent enough to see through that argument.

The toughest audience you ever have speaking about drugs is a bunch of teenage kids. Not only do they have most of the answers, but they think they know the ones they don't have. I'm against decriminalization because I believe we have to draw the line somewhere, and we have enough problems without legalizing marijuana. You say to decriminalize small amounts, but then where does that stop?

There are anti-drug people who paint marijuana as not only valueless, but evil. Do you think that we go too far in painting it?

I think we did that in the '30s. I think we did it in the '50s with my generation, when I was a kid. My parents told me horror stories about marijuana and they wouldn't have known marijuana if it had hit them in the face. Frankly, as you get a little older and get into service and see marijuana, you realize it will not make hair grow in the palms of your hand.

The Dangers of Marijuana

Some people say it's a benign drug, but I don't think it is because quite frankly, I [have] seen too many instances of people smoking and then they get thirsty and then they throw a little wine, maybe a quart or two. We talked to a fellow earlier today who almost blew up a laboratory because the ether and the marijuana and wine altogether. We don't know how many traffic accidents to attribute to it.

Plus in my experience I've seen people that have smoked for over 20 years and I've seen them become dull. Not everybody, by any chance, but a number of them and I can't account for any other thing they did in their life that made them dull, and these were not heavy smokers, but they smoked a joint or two a day. That's scary. That's not much. That's a couple of grams.

Was there a particular case that stands out as really affecting you?

It was a five-year investigation and involved individuals here and in Colorado and in New Mexico. Basically, they had a hothouse operation in southern Indiana that appeared to turn out about 7,000 to

8,000 plants every quarter. They owned at least two farms. One of a 119 acres and the other one of a 120, and they would set the plants out there and initially grow them in the hothouse and then set them out, harvest them and then transfer the dope out west.

Now, the investigation that we conducted indicated that these folks made $7 or $8 million in about a four year period of time. They admitted to making $1 million, so the truth is somewhere in between but $1 million is a lot of money for a part-time operation like that.

I'm concerned about the corruption that I have seen particularly in a couple of other areas in this country, not only to law enforcement, but to communities, in general, where the economic conditions are such that marijuana becomes a dominant force in that county or in that region and the police while a lot of times not involved are paid not to be involved if that makes any sense. They'll patrol this road for a month or two or for three or four days, or at night, and your business community, your banks, your merchants, they become a part of it because your children and citizens see them taking that money which they have to do to survive. It's not an easy answer, but it happens.

So there again, I'm against it. I've seen it happen. I see people get into it for one year of the growing season, "We're going to make the big win and quit." And they can't. The money's too easy, and eventually, those are the ones we catch. They have a saying in the marijuana business, "We're not millionaires, but we live like millionaires." Well, that's one way that we catch them, and they do it quite frequently—a lot of trips, lot of toys.

A Lucrative Enterprise

Tell me about the case of the two brothers—an architect and a lawyer.

Well, the two brothers had started on a small scale in Colorado. The architect was growing in his basement, he and his wife in his home in a suburb of Boulder. They made so much money with this fairly small crop of 300 or 400 plants, because it was an Afghani strain and that was new at the time. That must have been over ten years ago. That the next year they put in 3,000.

They jumped seedlings. They transported half of them to Nebraska and half of them out here. The brother that was an attorney had found a farmer that was in some financial difficulties, which a lot of people were about that time. The Reagan prosperity had busted out, and a lot of farmers had bought land high and crop prices had fallen, and the farmer agreed [to] plant a camouflage corn crop and basically nurture this marijuana crop—1,500 plants.

There were several participants, pickers and harvesters. This is formalized. It's almost [like] GM. People have different jobs and the low-level people make about $30,000 a year and the higher up in the organization you were, the more money you make.

Next year, they did it on a larger scale, but they had bad weather, and the guy that set the crops out didn't put the right herbicide in and they had a little agricultural disaster. So about that time, we'd become aware of it. There were search warrants and information that the Indiana State Police had developed out of the local community, and they got in one more crop and probably did fairly well with that probably. My guess is about 600 plants. And we were able to arrest them.

There were initially 16 people indicted. Seven of them pled guilty. Nine went to trial. The trial took nine weeks. We had offered a plea bargain of sentences from ten years down to three. They took, what we call the constitutional cruise, and when it was over the jury was out, I think, [for] four hours . . . and they got sentences up to 20 plus years, all guilty.

Now their contention is that they only made about $1 million, but by the money spent and the paper trail we were able to develop, we thought it was a lot more and there were fines levied particularly on the attorney for the amount of income. Their contention is that it all went for legal fees. I don't know.

An All-American Family

Was there something about the two brothers that struck you particularly?

Well, it was an interesting case in the organization and the loyalty that the people showed to each other. In a way, it was typical of marijuana cases in that these people were much better educated. The attorney was particularly hard to pin down because he was so well liked.

He was the epitome of a small-town lawyer. He did a lot of free work for people. He knew his job. He was respected in the profession, he was a good neighbor and people liked him. They're from a prominent Indiana family. The other brother [was] very likable. They had a lot of charisma and I became fairly well acquainted with them and I believe it's genuine. They're likable people. They're smarter than the average man and they were tougher to catch. It made the case very interesting. They had the money to hire the best legal talent, and got the best defense they could and then they went to prison.

It sounds like the all-American family.

They were the all-American boys. I had police information where they dabbled with drugs in junior high school, but they were the all-American boys. You would be very happy to sit down and talk to these people. They're interesting, they're engaging, they're sincere. They love their children. Smart. Nice. They broke the law and they knew better.

Should they have [received] the kind of sentence they got?

I think they should. It's one thing to catch somebody with 101 plants, which is generally the threshold for federal prosecution, but these people kept it up. They kept it up after we knew that we were investigating. I think they felt they could get away with it. I don't think they thought we could put the case together.

There were a lot of people in the community that shielded them out of misplaced loyalty or genuine loyalty and maybe dislike of the police. Who knows? Maybe they identified with the pirates more than they did with the Royal Navy. I don't know. That's a subject to itself. But should they have gotten the sentences? Yes, they should have, because that sends a message out that the people of Indiana will not tolerate this type of behavior.

Why should we say it's OK for a guy to make $1 million raising marijuana? Who are the end users of this marijuana? Marijuana is the threshold drug. It's the drug that most children start out with. In respect of what you were talking about earlier, is there really a difference between big marijuana and little marijuana? Remember there's two things about death and pregnancy, both being sort of final. Well, you could take the same view about marijuana. How much is enough? Too much.

Alternative Sentencing

What do you see happening now with federal sentencing and the mandatory minimums?

I think that the sentences are tougher, but I think the judges are more creative. I think you're seeing more alternative sentencing in marijuana cases. I think that if we trooped you in with a pound of crack, you would go to prison for 20 or 30 years. If we trooped you in with 100 pounds of marijuana, you'd probably be doing some community service down at the Girl's Club teaching girls how to make documentary films and everybody would be better off.

You wouldn't be in prison. You wouldn't be a burden on the taxpayer. You'd still be holding a job, hopefully paying taxes. It's a philosophical thing with them that I disagree with, but you'd still be contributing to the community. The second time we got you, good-bye.

How about the marijuana sentences? Are they proportionate to what violent criminals are getting?

I cannot see somebody in there doing eight years for marijuana and a rapist being set free. Anybody that abuses another human being, I have a certain loathing for. There's a disparity there, but that's not with law enforcement. We don't make the laws and we don't sentence the offenders. All we do is catch people. A lot of these people that we're talking about have only done one thing wrong. You know what that is? They got caught.

With your experience of working with growers, dealing with them, do you think that some kind of alternative sentencing in the marijuana area would work?

Oh, I think it does work. I think particularly on the first offense, but you got to understand, the first offense is not the first time they did it. They may have done it for ten years, it's just the first time we caught 'em.

But the judge has to sentence them from the facts in that case, and that's the law, and that's the way it should be and that's all the jury gets to hear if they go to trial. But it gets back to what I said earlier. A lot of these people have a skill. A lot of them have a legitimate job. And I believe they should be given a second chance. That's what America is. It's the land of the second chance. And these first time marijuana growers—give them a second chance. Now the second time around I kind of take a harsher viewpoint.

Examining the Facts of Each Case

The guy who is growing ten plants in his closet, what do you feel is appropriate for something like that?

Without knowing more facts on the case I couldn't tell you. What's his attitude? Was he violent to the police officers? Did he beat up his children when they protested the fact that he was growing marijuana? All these things have to figure in. If he's growing ten plants, let's say, just to make it a simple scenario, so he doesn't have to go out on the street, purchase marijuana, expose himself to the danger, I think the court would do well to consider alternative sentencing if there's an alternative there.

Does he have something to offer the community? Can he be punished and rehabilitated? Because, unfortunately, in this country we look for both. We never made up our mind. Do we want to punish these people or do we want to rehabilitate them? Almost 30 years in law enforcement, I have to believe some of them will never be rehabilitated. But quite a few can. And I've seen it happen and some times it's worth giving ten a break to rehabilitate one.

What was it that led you to advocate alternative sentencing?

I support alternative sentencing based on my experience with the marijuana traffickers in the Midwest. What I've seen the courts do here, in the Midwest, with alternative sentencing. Based on my past twenty years prior experience dealing with heroin and cocaine and amphetamine and LSD dealers—some of who did me physical damage and some who I did physical damage—because they're violent people and I quite frequently hear the argument that narcotics traffickers shouldn't be in prison with violent people. You better wake up because most of them are violent people. And they'll hurt 'ya.

Considering the Differences

But these marijuana growers and traffickers, even though they have a substantial capitol investment in here and are not violent towards us (the police) here, in some other states they are. I can only speak [from] my experience. But they're not violent toward the police. They're not violent toward their confederates. They're not violent towards the citizens. Now, they're different than the people that come out of Chicago or Cincinnati on the weekend to cut the fences and run their four wheels in here and pick as much as they can. These are people who have preserved these fields and do as little as possible to disturb the legitimate residents here. These are rural people and they mind their own business. They don't support crime and they were very supportive of us in our investigation. But they mind their own business. So that's the culture down here.

And these people are part of their culture and they take advantage of it. They have a place in the community and the courts. In one case I had 16 defendants in a marijuana conspiracy. Fourteen got alternative sentences. I agreed with that. It was Judge Sara Evans Barker in Indianapolis. She looked very much at what each individual had to offer the community and put them to work in the community.

Why put these people into a prison where they're going to get a master's or a Ph.D. in crime, which most of them haven't been exposed to anyway? They're just people growing marijuana. Give them a chance. Second time around? Sorry. No chance. First time, if they merit that break, give it to them. It's better for the community. Less people in the prison system. They're still out working and contributing. They're going to make an extra contribution whether it's picking up trash or teaching children or repairing toilets. That is a positive role. And I believe in that.

An Emotional Issue

Trigger point issues. Do you think that marijuana has become one of those?

It's an emotional issue, I think. It's right there with gays in the military and abortion. Everybody's got an opinion on it. When I started in law enforcement, the general opinion, particularly in the white middle class community was, "Marijuana? Send them to jail." Because they're probably black or Chicano to begin with. And it wasn't something that affected us. Now it touches everybody in America. And I don't think anybody doesn't have a family member in an extended family that hasn't been touched by it. So, there are some strong feelings.

A lot of times, I think they're irrational. I generally don't even talk to people about the subject. People find out that I was an agent, "What do you think of this?" I don't think about it very often. Because I don't know what I'm going to set off in these people and frankly I don't want to hear it. They don't, most cases, know as much about it as I do. They only know what happened to their nephew or their daughter. Or their son got beat up by the police. And maybe he did and maybe he didn't. I wasn't there, I don't know. But generally there's two sides to every question.

And you hear from people who say you've got to send this guy away.

Yes. There's not a particular middle ground. People just have very strong feelings about [it] and I don't think anybody's unemotional about marijuana. People a little younger than myself who particularly grew up, probably from the late '60s on, they tried it. And they in their cases got through it no fault, no foul. No harm. But yet, when you talk to them . . . I did a lot of public speaking when I was on the job, because I believe the public should be informed about this. And people would come up and say, "I do not want my children exposed to what I went through in the '60s, the '70s, the '80s." . . . Each one of them really sees it within the era that they were a teenager, in college or this, that and the other. And they have strong opinions. Most of them, most people who are parents are anti-marijuana. There is no middle ground for them. And that's why, I think, you see a lot of things going the way they are.

In Indiana and the Midwest, how are people balancing out in their opinion about marijuana right now?

Well, this is the law and order part of the country. It is a pleasure to work here. Law enforcement is held in probably higher esteem here than any place I've ever been. And government here is, generally, very clean. People are hard working. I would say that it is probably more conservative than any place I've been, but I haven't been everywhere so I don't know. Certainly, I know when I was in the Southwest, I think it was kind of rites of passage for people to smoke marijuana there. Up here, even though it grew so abundantly, I've met a lot of people who [have] never smoked marijuana. There's a different attitude here.

You think the fact that the people are different says something about marijuana itself?

No. Not about marijuana. [It] says something about the people that like marijuana, but marijuana is still a weed.

It sounds like what you're saying is you have one image as a person and as a law enforcement officer. Of people who use or deal with marijuana— you've come to have a slightly different view of that.

Probably. I entered into it with not really much of any impression of marijuana growers. Because I hadn't been around them that much. To me, they were just another class of law breakers. And then, in the five years that I ran the program and when I did so much work with them and worked the investigations, I came to see them as a different breed of cat. They're still criminals, but they don't have some of the characteristics of all the others that I dealt with in the 20 years previously. You'll find disagreements within the marijuana irradication community and law enforcement. There are guys in Northern California will say you're nuts. People out here shoot at us regularly. People in southern Oregon. Troopers in Kentucky and agents over there. They have a lot of violence there and they have a different culture. But we're talking about what I've experienced. And it's what I've experienced. They are different.

Marijuana policy and law really is a hard area to talk about for many people. Why is this issue so hard for people to discuss?

Well, because everybody has an opinion and it's based mostly on emotion rather than rationale. We decriminalized marijuana in this country in response with requests from other nations. At the turn of the [twentieth] century we were a source country for marijuana to North Africa and the Middle East. And they were under the Ottomans. They clamped down on marijuana production, hashish, hemp. And in return we signed treaties with them because we had a serious opiate and cocaine problem in this country from the Civil War on up. And we wanted to shut some of that traffic down.

An Objective Examination

All that was codified in the 1914 Harrison Narcotic Act, but it existed for a reason. It was there because at the time, it was a sincere problem. Whether we're not supplying marijuana to the Middle East, I doubt. But we're growing plenty for ourselves and it's better than what we import from Mexico and Colombia. So do we just roll over and play dead and say, "Hey, we give up?" That's [not] the American way. I do not believe that decriminalizing or legalizing is going to help in any way. The drug is still there. I do not care what people say. I talk to many people. It's an addictive drug. If not, physically, psychologically to make people have to have it every day. To get the heart started. To mellow out at the end of the day. I think it's a dangerous drug. I don't think it does any good. Period. It makes you feel better. Take your shoes off, put your feet in some hot water and that will help too.

But it's a tough issue. We have to look at the history. We have to go back in time as to why it happened. Like the '30s, we had gotten carried away with it. We got into that period of excess. Not only in the enforcement of the law but in the educational information that we put out on it. And that lasted through the '50s. The '60s came along and destroyed a lot of the myths about it. But, on the other hand, they have also because of the research done down at the University of Mississippi show that it's a carcinogen, there's no health value to it. [It has] 400 carcinogens in it. A lot more than tobacco does. And five times the potency. When you take that, coupled with the fact that marijuana burns at a higher temperature, it's dangerous. I see no benefit to it.

You're not for decriminalization or legalization. But it seems fair to say that you would like to see room made to step back and look at this whole area a little more objectively and calmly without so much emotion in the way we think about marijuana.

Let me put it to you this way. We probably spend more in this country to advertise coffee in one day than we do on marijuana research. We need more done in that area. The American public deserves the facts. What is this drug? The arguments are still, if you read the prior issue of *High Times*, some very good arguments for medical marijuana in there. But they're also shot with a couple of fallacies that I find. We need somebody people can believe in to actually say this is what it does, this is what it doesn't do, and try and take some of the emotion out of it. It has become too emotional an issue to too many people. But to say that I would ever be for decriminalization—there's no evidence that I've seen at this point in time that would make me go along with that.

ORGANIZATIONS TO CONTACT

The editors have compiled the following list of organizations concerned with the issues presented in this book. The descriptions are derived from materials provided by the organizations. All have publications or information available for interested readers. The list was compiled on the date of publication of the present volume; the information provided here may change. Be aware that many organizations take several weeks or longer to respond to inquiries, so allow as much time as possible.

Center for Substance Abuse Prevention (CSAP)
National Clearinghouse for Alcohol and Drug Information (NCADI)
PO Box 2345, Rockville, MD 20847-2345
(800) 729-6686 • fax: (301) 468-6433
e-mail: info@health.org • website: www.health.org

The CSAP leads U.S. government efforts to prevent substance abuse problems among Americans. Through the NCADI, the center provides the public with a wide variety of current information concerning substance abuse and drug policy. NCADI services include a staff equipped to respond to inquiries, a database of prevention-related materials, and the distribution of brochures, pamphlets, posters, and videotapes available through its toll-free number. Its publications include the bimonthly *Prevention Pipeline* and the booklet *Marijuana: Facts for Teens*. Publications in Spanish are also available.

Common Sense for Drug Policy
3220 N St. NW, #141, Washington, DC 20007
(703) 354-5694 • fax: (703) 354-5695
e-mail: info@csdp.org • website: www.csdp.org

The organization's mission is to educate the public about alternatives to current drug policy by disseminating research, hosting public forums, and informing the media. It also gives advice and technical assistance to allied organizations working to reform current drug policy. On its website, Common Sense provides access to news articles, data, and research concerning marijuana and other drugs. It also publishes the semiannual newspaper *Common Sense* and the book *Drug War Facts*, which includes a discussion of marijuana policy.

Drug Enforcement Administration (DEA)
Information Services Section (CPI)
2401 Jefferson Davis Hwy., Arlington, VA 22301
website: www.usdoj.gov/dea

Part of the U.S. Department of Justice, the DEA enforces the controlled substance laws and regulations of the United States, brings to justice those involved in the illegal cultivation, manufacture, or distribution of controlled substances, and supports nonenforcement programs aimed at reducing the availability of controlled substances on the domestic and international markets. Its publications include "Say It Straight: The Medical Myths of Marijuana," and "BC Bud: Growth of the Canadian Marijuana Trade."

DrugSense
PO Box 651, Porterville, CA 93258
(800) 266-5759

e-mail: MGreer@mapinc.org • website: www.drugsense.org

DrugSense is committed to heightening awareness of the damage caused by the war on drugs, informing the public of rational alternatives to the drug war, and helping organize citizens to bring about needed reforms. It promotes public debate and discussion of current drug policy and provides online and technical support to reform organizations. Through its Media Awareness Project, DrugSense maintains a database of current news and opinion articles about drugs and drug policy, including marijuana. The organization also publishes the newsletter *DrugSense Weekly*.

Families Against Mandatory Minimums (FAMM)
1612 K St. NW, Suite 1400, Washington, DC 20006
(202) 822-6700
e-mail: famm@famm.org • website: www.famm.org

Founded in 1991, FAMM is a national organization of citizens working to reform federal and state mandatory sentencing laws that remove judicial discretion, including those laws that deal with nonviolent drug-related offenses. The organization's efforts include educating the public and policy makers through media outreach, grassroots campaigns, and direct action. Its quarterly newsletter, the *FAMMGram*, features articles on sentencing, prisons, and legal news.

The Lindesmith Center–Drug Policy Foundation (TLC-DPF)
4455 Connecticut Ave. NW, Suite B-500, Washington, DC 20008-2328
(202) 537-5005 • fax: (202) 537-3007
e-mail: dc@drugpolicy.org • website: www.lindesmith.org

The TLC-DPF supports alternatives to the war on drugs, including a shift away from criminal justice policies and toward public health approaches to drug use and abuse. The organization provides grants for research on drug policy alternatives and hosts an international conference on drug policy reform. Its publications include the book *Marijuana Myths, Marijuana Facts: A Review of the Scientific Evidence*.

Marijuana Policy Project (MPP)
PO Box 77492, Capitol Hill, Washington, DC 20013
(202) 262-5747
e-mail: mpp@mpp.org • website: www.mpp.org

The MPP strives to minimize the harm associated with both the consumption and the prohibition of marijuana. The project's specific focus is on removing criminal penalties for marijuana use, particularly medicinal marijuana. Its activities include supporting legislation to allow states to determine their own policies concerning medical marijuana, gathering endorsements for legal reform from medical associations, and lobbying the National Institute on Drug Abuse to make marijuana available for FDA-approved research. The MPP also publishes the *Marijuana Policy Report*, a quarterly newsletter.

National Center on Addiction and Substance Abuse at Columbia University (CASA)
633 Third Ave., Floor 19, New York, NY 10017-6706
(212) 841-5200 • fax: (212) 956-8020
e-mail: mnakashi@casacolumbia.org • website: www.casacolumbia.org

CASA is a think tank composed of professionals from many disciplines—including business, communications, medicine, sociology, law, and law enforcement—whose goal is to inform Americans of the economic and social costs of substance abuse. The center performs studies on gateway drugs, legalization, and the impact of substance abuse. CASA's publications include the articles "Non-Medical Marijuana: Rite of Passage or Russian Roulette?" and "Cigarettes, Alcohol, Marijuana: Gateway to Illicit Drug Use."

National Drug Prevention League (NDPL)
16 S. Calvert St., Baltimore, MD 20202
(410) 385-9094 • fax: (410) 385-9096
e-mail: augustus@erols.com • website: www.ndpl.org

The NDPL is a coalition of national and regional organizations for the prevention of drug abuse. The league believes that drug abuse and addiction are at the root of the social, health, legal, and economic problems of families, communities, and the nation. Its goal is to foster a national resolve against drug abuse by promoting public awareness about prevention strategies and linking individual prevention efforts throughout the country. On its website, the NDPL provides access to national surveys and studies, congressional bills, and fact sheets concerning drug abuse.

National Institute on Drug Abuse (NIDA)
National Institutes of Health
6001 Executive Blvd., Room 5213, Bethesda, MD, 20892-9561
(301) 443-1124
e-mail: information@lists.nida.nih.gov • website: www.nida.nih.gov

Part of the National Institutes of Health, a research agency of the U.S. government, NIDA conducts scientific studies concerning the causes and effects of drug abuse. It distributes the results of its research to policy makers, practitioners, and the general public. Among NIDA's many publications are the books *Adolescent Marijuana Abusers and Their Families* and *Marijuana Effects on the Endocrine and Reproductive Systems*, the bimonthly newsletter *NIDA Notes*, and the educational series *Mind Over Matter*, which includes the magazine *The Brain's Response to Marijuana*.

National Organization for the Reform of Marijuana Laws (NORML)
1001 Connecticut Ave. NW, Suite 710, Washington, DC 20036
(202) 483-5500 • fax: (202) 483-0057
e-mail: norml@norml.org • website: www.norml.org

Since its founding in 1970, NORML has been the principal national advocate for ending the prohibition of marijuana. The organization lobbies state and federal legislators to permit the medical use of marijuana and to reject attempts to treat minor marijuana offenses more harshly. It publishes two quarterlies, the *NORML Legislative Bulletin* and the *NORML Leaflet*. On its website, NORML provides access to its weekly news bulletin, as well as studies and testimony concerning marijuana.

Office of National Drug Control Policy (ONDCP)
Drug Policy Information Clearinghouse
PO Box 6000, Rockville, MD 20849-6000
(800) 666-3332 • fax: (301) 519-5212
e-mail: ondcp@ncjrs.org • website: www.whitehousedrugpolicy.gov

The ONDCP establishes policies, priorities, and objectives for the nation's drug control program. The office's mission is to reduce the use, manufacturing, and trafficking of illicit drugs, drug-related crime and violence, and drug-related health consequences. Its website presents information on the nation's current drug control policies and facts and statistics on illicit drugs, as well as ONDCP publications such as "Maintaining Marijuana in Schedule I" and "Marijuana and Medicine: Assessing the Scientific Base."

Partnership for a Drug-Free America
405 Lexington Ave., Suite 1601, New York, NY 10174
(212) 922-1560 • fax: (212) 922-1570
website: www.drugfreeamerica.org

A coalition of professionals from the communications industry, the Partnership for a Drug-Free America is dedicated to reducing the demand for illegal drugs via media communication. Through its national anti-drug advertising campaign, the organization endeavors to change societal attitudes of support or toleration toward drug use. In addition, it conducts annual studies into the current attitudes of Americans toward drug abuse, which are available on its website. The organization publishes the monthly *Partnership Bulletin* and the biannual *Newsletter of the Partnership for a Drug-Free America*.

BIBLIOGRAPHY

Books

Dan Baum	*Smoke and Mirrors: The War on Drugs and the Politics of Failure.* Boston: Little, Brown, 1996.
Alan W. Bock	*Waiting to Inhale: The Politics of Medical Marijuana.* Santa Ana, CA: Seven Locks Press, 2000.
Dirk Chase Eldredge	*Ending the War on Drugs.* Bridgehampton, NY: Bridge Works, 1998.
Mark S. Gold	*Marijuana.* New York: Plenum, 1989.
Mike Gray	*Drug Crazy: How We Got into This Mess and How We Can Get Out.* New York: Random House, 1998.
Lester Grinspoon and James B. Bakalar	*Marijuana, The Forbidden Medicine.* New Haven, CT: Yale University Press, 1993.
Herbert Hendin, et al.	*Living High: Daily Marijuana Use Among Adults.* New York: Human Sciences Press, 1987.
Jack Herer	*Hemp and the Marijuana Conspiracy: The Emperor Wears No Clothes.* Van Nuys, CA: Hemp Pub., 1995.
Leslie L. Iversen	*The Science of Marijuana.* New York: Oxford University Press, 2000.
Janet E. Joy, Stanley J. Watson Jr., and John A. Benson Jr., eds.	*Marijuana and Medicine: Assessing the Science Base.* Washington, DC: National Academy Press, 1999.
Mark Kleiman	*Marijuana: Costs of Abuse, Costs of Control.* New York: Greenwood Press, 1989.
Mary Lynn Mathre, ed.	*Cannabis in Medical Practice: A Legal, Historical, and Pharmacological Overview of the Therapeutic Use of Marijuana.* Jefferson, NC: McFarland, 1997.
National Institute on Drug Abuse	*Marijuana: Facts Parents Need to Know.* Bethesda, MD: National Institute on Drug Abuse, 1998.
Robert Randall and Alice O'Leary	*Marijuana Rx: The Patient's Fight for Medicinal Pot.* New York: Thunders Mouth Press, 1998.
Ed Rosenthal	*Why Marijuana Should Be Legal.* New York: Thunders Mouth Press, 1996.
Larry Sloman	*Reefer Madness: The History of Marijuana in America.* New York: St. Martin's Griffin, 1998.
Substance Abuse and Mental Health Services Administration	*Tips for Teens: The Truth About Marijuana.* Rockville, MD: Center for Substance Abuse Prevention, 2000.
Lynn Zimmer and John P. Morgan	*Marijuana Myths, Marijuana Facts: A Review of the Scientific Evidence.* New York: Lindesmith Center, 1997.

Periodicals

Nurith C. Aizenmann "Smoked Out," *New Republic*, September 30, 1998.

George Annas "Reefer Madness: The Federal Response to California's Medical Marijuana Law," *New England Journal of Medicine*, June 1997. Available from Massachusetts Medical Society, 860 Winter St., Waltham, MA 02451-1413.

Richard Brookhiser "Lost in the Weed," *U.S. News & World Report*, January 13, 1997.

Jeffrey DeSimone "Is Marijuana a Gateway Drug?" *Eastern Economic Journal*, Spring 1998. Available from the Department of Economics, Iona College, New Rochelle, NY 10801-1890.

Ben Dickinson "What If Weed Is Exactly What You Need?" *Esquire*, October 1997.

Robert Dreyfuss "Another Victory for Medical Marijuana," *Rolling Stone*, May 13, 1999.

Kathleen Fackelmann "Marijuana on Trial: Is Marijuana a Dangerous Drug or a Valuable Medicine?" *Science News*, March 22, 1997.

Sarah Ferguson "The Battle for Medical Marijuana," *Nation*, January 6, 1997.

Erika Fortgang "Is Pot Bad for You? Six Questions Answered," *Rolling Stone*, March 4, 1999.

Wayne Hall and Nadia Solowij "Adverse Effects of Cannabis," *Lancet*, November 14, 1998. Available from the Lancet Publishing Group, 655 Avenue of the Americas, New York, NY 10010, or at www.thelancet.com/journal/vol352/iss9140/contents.

Richard B. Heyman and Rina M. Anglin "Marijuana: A Continuing Concern for Pediatricians," *Pediatrics*, October 1999. Available from American Academy of Pediatricians, PO Box 927, Elk Grove, IL 60009-0927.

John R. Hubbard and Sharone E. Franco "Marijuana: Medical Implications," *American Family Physician*, December 1999. Available from 11400 Tomahawk Creek Pkwy., Leawood, KS 66211-2672.

Phil Jenkins "Field of Opportunity," *Canadian Geographic*, March/April 1999.

J.P. Kassier "Federal Foolishness and Marijuana," *New England Journal of Medicine*, June 1997.

J. Maira "Marijuana: The Public Wants to Drag the Camel into the Tent," *Alcoholism and Drug Abuse Weekly*, February 10, 1997. Available from Manisses Communications Group, 208 Governor St., Providence, RI 02906.

Brian Preston "Vancouver's Pot Experiment," *Rolling Stone*, April 2, 1998.

Wayne J. Roques "Medical Marijuana: Compassion or Cruelty?" *Alcoholism and Drug Abuse Weekly*, November 17, 1997.

Ryan H. Sager	"Grass Roots: The Progress of Medical Marijuana," *National Review*, November 8, 1999.
Craig Savoye	"Move to Legalize Hemp Grows in Heartland," *Christian Science Monitor*, February 13, 2001.
Chef Scerra and Keith Green	"Marijuana: An Ineffective Way to Control Glaucoma," *Ophthalmology Times*, January 15, 1999. Available from Advanstar Communications, 7500 Old Oak Blvd., Cleveland, OH 44130.
Eric Schlosser	"The Politics of Pot: A Government in Denial," *Rolling Stone*, March 4, 1999.
Charles R. Schwenk	"Marijuana and Job Performance: Comparing the Major Streams of Research," *Journal of Drug Issues*, Fall 1998. Available from Florida State University, School of Criminology and Criminal Justice, Journal of Drug Issues, PO Box 66696, Tallahassee, FL 32313-6696.
Donna E. Shalala	"Say 'No' to Legalization of Marijuana," *Wall Street Journal*, August 18, 1995.
Steve Sussman and Alan W. Stacy	"Marijuana Use: Current Issues and New Research Directions," *Journal of Drug Issues*, Fall 1996.
Andrew Peyton Thomas	"Marijuana and Mea Culpas," *American Enterprise*, May/June 1997.

INDEX

McCoy, Burl, 76–77
McDonough, James R.
  on delivery systems, 105–106,
    114–15
  on medical research, 107–11
  on state laws vs. federal regulation,
    111–13
McDougal, Jeanette, 76–77
megestrol acetate, 96
Mellon, Andrew, 68
memory, 23, 35, 89
  see also brain
Mill, John Stuart, 51
Minnesota, 74
Missouri, 71
Monitoring the Future Survey, 38, 65
Monroe, Judy, 33–35
Monson, David, 73
Montana, 73, 74
Moran, Carolyn, 71
Morgan, John P., 30–32
Morris, David, 76
multiple sclerosis, 94–95

Nader, Ralph, 74–75
Nahas, Gabriel, 21
NAIHC, 74
naloxone, 29
National Academy of Sciences (NAS),
  20, 52
  see also Institute of Medicine
National Commission on Marihuana
  and Drug Abuse, 52
National Conference on Marijuana
  Use (1995), 62
National Household Survey, 38
National Institute on Drug Abuse
  (NIDA), 28, 58, 96
  anti-drug campaign of, 30
  research cancelled by, 15, 16
  study on driving under influence,
    34
National Institutes of Health (NIH),
  85, 94, 96, 106
National Organization for the Reform
  of Marijuana Laws (NORML), 47,
  57, 76, 84
Native Americans, 74–75
nausea, 17, 18, 85, 94, 107
  from Crohn's disease, 122
  delta-9-tetrahydrocannabinol for,
    95
Navarro, Miguel, 27
needle-exchange programs, 79
Newkirk, Gary, 101–104

New Mexico, 73, 74
New York Times (newspaper), 38, 97,
  106
New York Times Magazine, 43
Nixon, Richard, 52, 128
North American Industrial Hemp
  Alliance (NAIHC), 70, 71
North Dakota, 67, 73

Oakland Cannabis Buyers'
  Cooperative, 83–84
Office of National Drug Control
  Policy, 39–40, 83
Ohio, 111
Olympic Games, 50
"On Liberty" (Mill), 51
Our Bodies and How We Live
  (Blaisdell), 39, 43
overdosing, 23

pain management, 85, 89
paraphernalia, 21–22
Parent Resouce Institute for Drug
  Education (PRIDE), 64–65
parents
  anti-drug campaigns targeted to,
    42–43
  illegal activities of, 148–49
  medicating children with
    marijuana, 122–26
  recognizing addiction in children,
    117–21, 124
Partnership for a Drug-Free America,
  83, 85
  advertisements by, 22, 40, 41
  "gateway" theory of, 30
Pennekamp, Peter, 79, 80
Perez, D.S., 54–56
Peron, Dennis
  California Proposition 215
    campaign of, 127–30
  on future of Cannabis Cultivators'
    Club, 132–33
Peterson, Linda
  on California Proposition 215
    campaign, 127–30
  on future of Cannabis Cultivators'
    Club, 132–33
  on life of Peron, 130–32
Pine Ridge Reservation (South
  Dakota), 75
Pope, Harrison G., Jr., 41
Popular Mechanics (magazine), 68
potency. See tetrahydrocannabinol
"Principles of Responsible Cannabis